WC SISVAN 2010

D1325181

Introduction to Pandemic Influenza

WITHDRAWN

This book is for Karen, Paul, and both of our families.
In memory of Rob Sellwood (1947–1998).

Introduction to Pandemic Influenza

Edited by

Jonathan Van-Tam

MBE BMedSci(Hons) BMBS DM FFPH FRSPH
Professor of Health Protection, University of Nottingham, UK

Chloe Sellwood

BSc(Hons) PhD FRSPH
Pandemic Flu Lead, London Strategic Health Authority, National Health Service,
London, UK

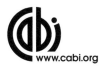
www.cabi.org

CABI is a trading name of CAB International

CABI Head Office	CABI North American Office
Nosworthy Way	875 Massachusetts Avenue
Wallingford	7th Floor
Oxfordshire OX10 8DE	Cambridge, MA 02139
UK	USA
Tel: +44 (0)1491 832111	Tel: +1 617 395 4056
Fax: +44 (0)1491 833508	Fax: +1 617 354 6875
E-mail: cabi@cabi.org	E-mail: cabi-nao@cabi.org
Website: www.cabi.org	

© CAB International 2010. All rights reserved. No part of this publication may be reproduced in any form or by any means, electronically, mechanically, by photocopying, recording or otherwise, without the prior permission of the copyright owners.

A catalogue record for this book is available from the British Library, London, UK.

Library of Congress Cataloging-in-Publication Data

Introduction to pandemic influenza / edited by Jonathan Van-Tam and Chloe Sellwood.
        p. cm. -- (Modular texts.)
    Includes bibliographical references and index.
    ISBN 978-1-84593-578-8 (alk. paper)

    1. Influenza--Epidemiology. 2. Influenza--Prevention. I. Van-Tam, Jonathan. II. Sellwood, Chloe. III. C.A.B. International. IV. Series: Modular texts.
    [DNLM: 1. Disease Outbreaks. 2. Influenza, Human--epidemiology. 3. Communicable Disease Control. 4. Disaster Planning. 5. Public Health Practice. WC 515 I618 2010]

    RA644.I6I585 2010
    614.5'18--dc22

                                        2009022097

ISBN: 978 1 84593 578 8 (paperback)
ISBN: 978 1 84593 625 9 (hardback)

Typeset by SPi, Pondicherry, India.
Printed and bound in the UK by Cambridge University Press, Cambridge.

The paper used for the text pages in this book is FSC certified. The FSC (Forest Stewardship Council) is an international network to promote responsible management of the world's forests.

Contents

Library and eLearning Centre
Gartnavel General Hospital

Contributors

Shukhrat Aripov, *Program Officer, Eastern Europe and Central Asia Team, The Global Fund To Fight AIDS, Tuberculosis and Malaria, Chemin de Blandonnet 8, 1214 Vernier, Geneva, Switzerland; Shukhrat.Aripov@TheGlobalFund.org*

Emily Collins, *MCIPR Regional Communications Manager, UK Health Protection Agency, London Region, 7th Floor, 330 High Holborn, London WC1V 7PP, UK; emily.collins@hpa.org.uk*

Joanne Enstone, *Research Coordinator for Influenza Studies, University of Nottingham, Epidemiology and Public Health, Clinical Sciences Building, Nottingham City Hospital, Hucknall Road, Nottingham NG5 1PB, UK; joanne.enstone@nottingham.ac.uk*

Elaine M. Gadd, *Honorary Professor, School of Law, Queen Mary University of London.*

Peter G. Grove, *Senior Principal Analyst, Department of Health, Health Protection Analytical Team.*

Ravindra K. Gupta, *Clinical Research Fellow, University College London, Windeyer Building, 46 Cleveland Street, London W1T 4JF, UK; rebmrag@ucl.ac.uk*

Lars R. Haaheim, *formerly Professor and Head, Influenza Centre, The Gade Institute, University of Bergen, Myrdalskogen 95, N-5117 Ulset, Norway; lars.haaheim@gades.uib.no*

David Hagen, *Consultant in Communicable Disease Control, Sussex & Surrey Health Protection Unit, Health Protection Agency, West Sussex Office, 9 College Lane, Chichester PO19 6FX, UK; david.hagen@hpa.org.uk*

Luc Hessel, *Executive Director, Policy Affairs Europe, Sanofi Pasteur MSD, 8 rue Jonas Salk, 69367 Lyon Cedex 07, France; lhessel@spmsd.com*

Lance C. Jennings, *Clinical Associate Professor, Canterbury Health Laboratories & Department of Pathology, University of Otago, Christchurch, New Zealand and Virology Section, Canterbury Health Laboratories, PO Box 151, Cnr Hagley Ave & Tuam St, Christchurch 8011, New Zealand; lance.jennings@cdhb.govt.nz*

Howard Needham, *Scientific Liaison Officer, European Centre for Disease Prevention and Control (ECDC), SE-171 83 Stockholm, Sweden; howard.needham@ecdc.europa.eu*

Angus Nicoll, *Senior Expert, Influenza Coordination, European Centre for Disease Prevention and Control (ECDC), SE-171 83 Stockholm, Sweden; angus.nicoll@ecdc.europa.eu*

Richard Puleston, *Associate Professor of Health Protection, University of Nottingham and Honorary Consultant Health Protection Agency, Epidemiology and Public Health, Clinical Sciences Building, Nottingham City Hospital, Hucknall Road, Nottingham NG5 1PB, UK; richard.puleston@nottingham.ac.uk*

Chloe Sellwood, *Pandemic Flu Lead, London Strategic Health Authority, NHS London, Southside, 105 Victoria Street, London SW1E 6QT, UK; chloe.sellwood@ london.nhs.uk*

John Simpson, *Regional Director and Head of Emergency Response Department, Centre for Emergency Preparedness and Response, Health Protection Agency, Porton Down, Salisbury SP4 0JG, UK; john.simpson@hpa.org.uk*

Jonathan Van-Tam, MBE, *Professor of Health Protection, University of Nottingham, Epidemiology and Public Health, Clinical Sciences Building, Nottingham City Hospital, Hucknall Road, Nottingham NG5 1PB, UK; jvt@nottingham.ac.uk*

Editor Biographies

Jonathan Van-Tam, MBE BMedSci(Hons) BMBS DM FFPH FRSPH, is Professor of Health Protection at the University of Nottingham. He graduated in medicine in 1987 and after several years of clinical work, completed academic training in epidemiology and public health, with a special interest in influenza that now spans almost 20 years. He brings a wealth of experience to this book including formative training in influenza under the mentorship of Professor Karl Nicholson, and private sector experience with two major pharmaceutical companies (both manufacturers of neuraminidase inhibitors) and a large European vaccines company. He returned to the public sector in 2007 and was Head of the Health Protection Agency, Pandemic Influenza Office during the most frenetic period of UK preparedness activity from 2004 to 2007. He has served as both Temporary Adviser and Short Term Consultant to the World Health Organization (WHO) regarding pandemic preparedness on numerous occasions, and has also undertaken related scientific work for the European Centre for Disease Prevention and Control (ECDC). He is a serving member of the UK national Scientific Pandemic Influenza Committee (SPI), its Clinical Countermeasures Sub-Group and a member of the newly formed UK Scientific Advisory Group for Emergencies (SAGE).

Chloe Sellwood, BSc(Hons) PhD FRSPH, works for the UK National Health Service (NHS) Strategic Health Authority (SHA) in London where she is the Pandemic Influenza Lead. She graduated in biochemistry in 1998 and completed a PhD in plant biochemistry in 2001. Her experience in pandemic preparedness ranges from international to local level, and encompasses both scientific and operational aspects. She spent over 7 years at the Health Protection Agency Centre for Infections, including 3 years as the Senior Scientist and Coordinator of the Pandemic Influenza Office from 2005 to 2008. She has worked with the WHO and the ECDC on international consultations, as well as on secondment to the Department of Health in England's Pandemic Influenza Preparedness Programme. In her current role she is responsible for the strategic overview of influenza pandemic preparedness within the NHS in London.

Foreword

In 2006 the Chief Medical Officer of England, Sir Liam Donaldson, wrote 'a pandemic of human influenza is on the horizon: the question is not whether it will arrive but when'. This belief, shared by influenza experts worldwide, explains the unprecedented importance of pandemic preparedness in terms of the global public health agenda. This book, prepared by experts under the authoritative editorship of Professor Jonathan Van-Tam and Dr Chloe Sellwood, is therefore both timely and important.

The editors and authors have worked closely together on UK and international pandemic preparedness for the last several years, during which ideas on pandemic preparedness evolved rapidly. For example, in 2004 the notion of 'pre-pandemic vaccination' was purely theoretical, yet now in 2009 one such 'pre-pandemic vaccine' (human A/H5N1 vaccine) is already licensed and several more will almost certainly follow over the next 12 months. Modelling studies performed in the last few years have revolutionized thinking about how antiviral drugs and vaccines might be used to greatest effect during a pandemic. The intense activity of the last 5 years has also exposed deficiencies and previous complacency related to our understanding of the mechanisms of influenza transmission and the effectiveness of simple interventions such as face masks and good respiratory/hand hygiene.

Pandemic influenza creates a whole-of-society problem that requires an equally broad response. Traditional infectious disease textbooks – even those devoted exclusively to influenza – do not cover issues such as modelling, pandemic response ethics, communications, business continuity and public health countermeasures. Information on these key areas of pandemic preparedness is also difficult to assimilate from peer-reviewed journals aimed at specialist audiences. In addition, as influenza pandemic preparedness has expanded in breadth and depth, it has engaged large numbers of public health practitioners who, by their own admission, are not influenza experts. Similarly, professional planners and local authority officials without any specific medical or clinical training must also rapidly get to grips with the subject. This is especially true at regional and local levels.

As requests for lectures and presentations increased rapidly, the authors recognized a pressing need for a new kind of textbook that would assist 'non-expert' public health professionals and the well-qualified lay-person to gain a rapid overview of pandemic influenza. This book is aimed at meeting such a need, and in my view fulfils it exceptionally well, giving the reader a good foundation in the broad range of subjects covered by the umbrella term 'influenza pandemic preparedness'.

The book comprises 16 chapters written by experts with real-life experience of their subjects. It provides a comprehensive overview of pandemic influenza with strong emphasis on practical topics related to preparedness, including pharmaceutical and public health countermeasures, policy issues, infection control, communication, ethics and modern bio-mathematical modelling. It is highly relevant to public health professionals and local authority officials involved in pandemic preparedness in both developing and developed nations, and will also be valuable to students of public health-related subjects. I congratulate the authors and editors on their achievement and believe it will prove an important learning resource for people in many countries as the world continues to prepare for the next influenza pandemic.

Novel Influenza A/H1N1 Virus in North America

As this book goes to press, another unexpected twist to the story of human influenza is unfolding, prompting a rapid extension to this foreword, although sadly there has been no time to supplement the main text. In the space of less than 1 week in late April 2009, the World Health Organization global pandemic alert level was raised from Phase 3 to Phase 5 based on revised definitions that came into force at around the same time, and which are detailed in Chapter 4 of this book. Phase 5 denotes sustained community-level outbreaks of an animal or human–animal influenza reassortant virus in two or more countries in one WHO region. Thus, the world is once again poised on the brink of an influenza pandemic – potentially the first one of the 21st century. The intensive pandemic planning of the past 5 years may be about to be put to the test across the globe and we are again reminded that influenza A/H5N1 (bird flu) is not the only novel virus with pandemic potential.

The present crisis began in March 2009 when Mexico experienced an extensive outbreak of an initially unknown respiratory illness; the epidemic curve began to accelerate in mid-April and had largely returned to baseline by late May. Although epidemiological data were limited at first (reinforcing the need for robust surveillance as outlined in Chapter 1), some illness was reportedly severe and deaths occurred. Because of difficulties in defining denominators, estimates of case fatality and hospitalization rates are not totally reliable at this stage. On 23 April 2009 the USA confirmed a small number of human influenza A infections in its southern states, mainly those bordering Mexico, that could not be sub-typed. These viruses were later analysed to be a novel reassortant A/H1N1 containing six genes from a North American swine flu virus and two new ones from a Eurasian swine virus. At least some of the Mexican cases were then subsequently linked to the same virus. A Public Health Emergency of International Concern (PHEIC) was declared by Mexico on 25 April 2009, WHO Phase 4 was triggered on 27 April, followed by Phase 5 on 29 April 2009.

At the present time, in early June 2009, the novel A/H1N1 virus has now affected over 65 countries across all major continents of the world (under-ascertainment remains possible in many countries). It therefore seems highly likely that a pandemic will be declared in the near future. Although the number of confirmed cases in most declared countries is currently small (c.500 or less), being driven initially by international travel and somewhat limited community spread, thousands of cases are now apparent in Canada, Mexico (where the epidemic has already passed its peak) and the USA where there is, or has been, evidence of widespread and sustained community transmission.

Thus far the clinical severity of the illness has been generally mild. However, a small proportion of severe illness including deaths (case fatality rate ≈0.2%) and hospitalizations (4–6%) is apparent from both US and Mexican data, predominantly in younger adults, many with underlying co-morbidities, including pregnancy. The illness features are similar to seasonal influenza but with a greater proportion of cases reporting diarrhoea, and the virus is so far sensitive to both licensed neuraminidase inhibitors, but resistant to adamantanes. In epidemiological terms, disease activity has been far greater among children and young adults than the elderly, with several large school-based outbreaks described. At the present time R_0 has been estimated to be between 1.4 and 1.6 in Mexico, higher in children than adults, but overall far lower outside North America.

As we enter the period of the northern hemisphere summer, there is great uncertainty about whether virus activity will decline as ambient temperatures increase, and whether there will then be a resurgent 'second wave' in autumn/winter 2009 as happened in 1918 (this seems likely). Although the novel A/H1N1 virus appears to provoke a generally mild illness at the present time, this is not assured for the future, and it should be remembered that in 1918 the severity of disease due to an A/H1N1 pandemic virus increased markedly during the second, autumn wave. Much crucial new epidemiological, clinical and virological information will be gained from close scrutiny of the virus and those who become infected with it during the southern hemisphere winter season, which is just beginning.

The emergence of A/H1N1 in Mexico, and its rapid spread across continents, underscores the need for relevant training material to ensure common understanding and wide participation in the global response to this virus and to other influenza viruses with human pandemic potential, such as avian influenza A/H5N1. Congratulations to the authors, editors and publishers of this book for creating a crucial international resource at a time when it is so clearly needed.

Sir Gordon Duff FRCP FMedSci FRSE
Florey Professor of Molecular Medicine, University of Sheffield, UK
(Chairman, Scientific Pandemic Influenza Advisory Committee (SPI), UK)

Further Reading

Centers for Disease Control and Prevention (2009) Hospitalized patients with novel influenza A (H1N1) virus infection – California, April–May, 2009. *Morbidity and Mortality Weekly Report* 58 (Early Release), 1–5; available at http://www.cdc.gov/mmwr/preview/mmwrhtml/mm58e0518a1.htm?s_cid=rr58e0518a1_e (accessed June 2009).

Centers for Disease Control and Prevention (2009) Novel influenza A (H1N1) virus infections in three pregnant women – United States, April–May 2009. *Morbidity and Mortality Weekly Report* 58, 497–500; available at http://www.cdc.gov/mmwr/preview/mmwrhtml/mm5818a3.htm (accessed June 2009).

Donaldson, L. (2006) A pandemic on the horizon. *Journal of the Royal Society of Medicine* 99, 222–225.

Fraser, C., Donnelly, C.A., Cauchemez, S., Hanage, W.P., Van Kerkhove, M.D., Hollingsworth, T.D., Griffin, J., Baggaley, R.F., Jenkins, H.E., Lyons, E.J., Jombart, T., Hinsley, W.R., Grassly, N.C., Balloux, F., Ghani, A.C., Ferguson, N.M., Rambaut, A., Pybus, O.G., Lopez-Gatell, H., Apluche-Aranda, C.M., Chapela, I.B., Zavala, E.P., Guevara, D.M., Checchi, F., Garcia, E., Hugonnet, S. and Roth, C.; The WHO Rapid Pandemic Assessment Collaboration (2009) Pandemic potential of a strain of influenza A (H1N1): early findings. *Science* 324, 1557–1561.

Novel Swine-Origin Influenza A (H1N1) Virus Investigation Team (2009) Emergence of a novel swine-origin influenza A (H1N1) virus in humans. *New England Journal of Medicine* 360, 2605–2615; available at http://content.nejm.org/cgi/content/full/NEJMoa0903810. Erratum at http://content.nejm.org/cgi/content/full/NEJMx090021v1 (accessed June 2009).

World Health Organization (2009) Considerations for assessing the severity of an influenza pandemic. *Weekly Epidemiological Record* 84, 197–212; available at http://www.who.int/wer/2009/wer8422.pdf (accessed June 2009).

World Health Organization (2009) *Epidemic and Pandemic Alert and Response (EPR). Influenza A(H1N1) – update 43.* http://www.who.int/csr/don/2009_06_03/en/index.html (accessed June 2009).

World Health Organization (2009) *Human infection with new influenza A (H1N1) virus: clinical observations from Mexico and other affected countries. Weekly Epidemiological Record* 84, 185–196; available at http://www.who.int/wer/2009/wer8421.pdf (accessed June 2009).

Acknowledgements

We realized from the outset that in order to create the best possible textbook, we would need the help and assistance of people who are not only recognized as experts in their field, but who are also excellent communicators and teachers. We thank all of the contributing authors who have dedicated their valuable time and expertise to this project and endured many months of working with us; without them, the task of assembling this volume would have been considerably more daunting. So much of the knowledge about pandemic preparedness is held within the new 'international fellowship' of pandemic planners with whom we have interacted over several intense years. We thank these colleagues, too numerous to mention individually, for the facts and wisdom they have imparted. Such a book could not have been produced without also drawing on the published outputs from the World Health Organization, the European Centre for Disease Prevention and Control and other organizations that have made sustained efforts towards international pandemic preparedness over a number of years.

The opinions expressed by the editors and authors contributing to this book do not necessarily reflect the opinions of the institutions or organizations with which they are affiliated or by whom they are employed.

JVT and CS

Glossary

Adjuvant. A compound or agent deliberately added to a vaccine in order to increase the antibody response while having few, if any, direct effects of its own. Especially useful in situations where a 'plain' vaccine produces only a modest antibody response; or for public health reasons, the available antigen needs to be eked out to produce more doses for a larger number of people (known as an 'antigen sparing' strategy).

Adverse effects/Adverse events. Unwanted side-effects caused by a medicine (or vaccine).

Antigenic drift. Changes to viral antigens, which occur through a process of random genetic mutation. Such changes are relatively frequent in RNA viruses such as influenza. Antigenic drift drives the production of new annual seasonal influenza vaccines, because pre-existing antibodies become poorly matched against the new drifted virus.

Antigenic shift. Reassortment of two or more influenza virus subtypes that causes a phenotypic change and the formation of a new subtype having a mixture of the surface antigens of the original viruses (e.g. A/H1N1+A/H3N2=A/H1N2).

Antiviral resistance. Development of reduced drug effectiveness (e.g. antivirals) in curing a disease (e.g. influenza), often due to reduced ability to neutralize the pathogen. This phenomenon may be caused by antigenic drift, natural selection or drug pressure (widespread use of the drug causes frequent exposure of the organism to the drug and accelerates the emergence of resistant variants).

Asymptomatic infections. Infections that do not cause any symptoms (note: some asymptomatic patients may still be infectious to others).

Booster (dose). Re-exposure to an immunizing antigen (usually by means of an additional dose of vaccine) after a period of time, that raises immunity (antibodies) against that antigen back up to protective levels, sometimes enhancing these above the levels produced by the primary immunization.

Boundary issues. Issues connected with deciding how to divide populations into those receiving and not receiving a treatment or intervention, e.g. who is and who is not a social contact of a case and therefore eligible for prophylaxis, who is and who is not a front-line healthcare worker.

Business continuity planning (BCP). The development and testing of a plan (the business continuity plan) for organizational continuity of critical functions during an incident or period of extended disruption, including the post-incident recovery phase and return to normality within a predefined time.

Case fatality rate (CFR). The proportion of people who become ill with symptoms and subsequently die as a consequence of their infection.

Cell-mediated immunity (CMI). Immunity that is not dependent on the raising of antibodies.

Clade. A group of influenza virus strains from a single common ancestor (analogous to a human family, tribe or clan); there are at least ten clades within the influenza A/H5N1 subtype. Important in relation to pre-pandemic vaccination and cross-protective immunity (see below).

Clinical attack rate (CAR). The proportion of a population who will become ill with symptoms over the period of a pandemic (note: not all at precisely the same time).

Cohorted care. A method of care used in situations where infection control is critical. Patients with the same illness are separated from patients who do not have the illness. Staff are also separated into those caring for 'ill' patients and those caring for 'not ill' patients.

Co-morbidity. A pre-existing chronic illness or condition, usually used to define medical conditions that are known to place the individual at greater risk from influenza complications, hospitalizations and death.

Cross-protective immunity. A situation where immunity to one antigen (stimulated by vaccination or wild infection) provides partial or complete protection against a range of similar antigens, e.g. when a vaccine containing A/H5N1 clade 2 antigens is capable of providing partial or complete protection against clade 1 and clade 3 viruses of the same A/H5N1 subtype. Very important in relation to pre-pandemic vaccination.

Cytokine storm. Pro-inflammatory proteins known as cytokines and chemokines which activate T-cells and macrophages can be released in response to severe infection. If released in large enough quantity (a cytokine 'storm'), these have the effect of producing an intense immune response, which is in itself potentially life-threatening. Cytokine storm is implicated in the severe manifestation of some human A/H5N1 infections and may have played a role in severe human A/H1N1 infections in young adults during the 1918–19 pandemic, when paradoxically a young and vigorous immune system may have been disadvantageous.

Defence in depth. Combinations of pandemic countermeasures that, when taken together, will most likely be more effective than single measures, and offer assurance that if some measures fail altogether, others will 'hold'. Also known as 'layered interventions' or 'layered containment' (although it is arguable whether pandemic influenza can ever be truly contained).

Double-blind placebo-controlled trial. A double-blind placebo-controlled trial is a way of carrying out an experiment that is designed to remove subjective bias on the part of the researcher and subject, where allocation to treatment is on the basis of chance alone and neither knows who belongs to the control or experimental groups. The use of a placebo in the comparison group ensures that the behavioural effect of being treated is the same in both groups.

Effectiveness. The capability of a treatment or countermeasure to produce the desired effect under 'real life' conditions, e.g. use of facemasks by people in their own homes.

Efficacy. The capability of a treatment or countermeasure to produce the desired effect under 'ideal' or perfectly controlled conditions, e.g. use of facemasks by supervised, motivated volunteers in a quarantine unit study.

Emergency preparedness. A process of dealing with and avoiding risks, through preparing for an emergency before it occurs; this often includes exercising the response.

Endemic. When a disease is endemic (from the Greek *en* meaning 'in' and *demos* meaning 'people'), it means that the illness or infection is persistently present in a certain fraction of a population group. For influenza the term endemic is not especially applicable, as the virus usually afflicts a population group in a wave of acute infections and thereafter returns to baseline in a classical epidemic pattern (see below).

Enzootic. Equivalent of endemic, but a term applied to animals, e.g. avian influenza is enzootic for some bird species in many areas in South-east Asia. Unfortunately, even in highly prestigious scientific journals the A/H5N1 virus in birds is said to be endemic; the correct term is of course enzootic.

Epidemic. A sudden surge of new influenza cases rising sharply above baseline, before returning again. For a given geographical location, an influenza epidemic period typically lasts about 6 to 10 weeks, the incidence rate taking a bell-shaped form. Epidemic is derived from the Greek meaning 'upon people'.

Epizootic. Equivalent of epidemic, but a term applied to animals.

Exercise. A process of testing and refining plans and preparedness through simulation. In the context of pandemic influenza, simulating the event and testing what might happen by way of organizational response/reaction.

Haemagglutinin. A glycosylated surface protein on the influenza virus that initiates infection by binding to receptors on the host cell.

Infection control. A collection of measures intended to reduce the risk of transmission from an infected person to uninfected persons (e.g. hand and respiratory hygiene, masks and respirators, disinfection). A term traditionally used in health and social care settings but in a pandemic has far wider applicability.

Influenza-like illness (ILI). Term used to describe a syndrome commonly associated with influenza infection. It is well recognized that the syndrome is fairly non-specific and without laboratory confirmation may inadvertently capture many other acute respiratory virus infections; however, ILI becomes much more predictive of true influenza at times of known virus activity, e.g. during epidemic and pandemic periods.

Interoperability. An imprecise term applied to how countries and organizations might plan to act before and during a pandemic in a way that is compatible with each other, or at least does not produce conflicting ideas and responses.

Layered interventions (or layered containment). Combinations of countermeasures that when taken together will be even more effective than single interventions, and offer assurance that if some measures fail altogether, others will 'hold'; also known as 'defence in depth'.

Live attenuated influenza vaccine (LAIV). A type of influenza vaccine made with virus that has not undergone a process of inactivation (i.e. has not been killed); instead the virus has been cultured to introduce mutations that weaken the virus, preserving its basic ability to produce an antibody response but without making the recipient ill.

M2-channel blockers. Antiviral drugs specific to influenza, which work by preventing the influenza virus from inserting its RNA into the host cell nucleus, e.g. amantadine or rimantadine.

Magistral. Referring to a drug or medicine: formulated extemporaneously or for a special purpose, e.g. Tamiflu® magistral formulation and emergency reconstition.

Mathematical modelling. Techniques using broad knowledge of the system under investigation to construct simplified, idealized versions (models) that can then be analysed in detail using complex mathematical techniques to predict what might happen given certain assumptions. Extensively used in pandemic preparedness to scope the possible extent of spread of disease and the effects of interventions.

Mock-up pandemic influenza vaccine. A vaccine that contains any influenza virus subtype to which man has not yet been exposed, with vaccine composition and manufacturing methods that are identical to those that will eventually be used for future pandemic influenza vaccine. This product is then licensed in advance. At the last moment when a pandemic virus is identified, a suitable antigen (vaccine seed virus) is decided upon and vaccine production begins without the need for a further lengthy licensing process.

Monovalent vaccine. Types of influenza vaccine containing only one strain of influenza virus (e.g. a pandemic strain) as opposed to the three strains normally present in seasonal influenza vaccines.

Morbidity. Poor health, illness or disability falling short of death (mortality). In relation to influenza, the term is frequently used fairly loosely to describe significant illness, complications and hospitalizations.

Neuraminidase. A glycosylated surface protein on the influenza virus that allows newly made virions to detach from the infected host cell and spread to infect other cells.

Neuraminidase inhibitors. Antiviral drugs specific to influenza that bind to the influenza neuraminidase, thereby blocking the release of newly formed virus particles from infected host cells.

Non-pharmaceutical interventions. Measures of influenza control that do not include pharmaceutical products such as vaccines and drugs.

Nosocomial infection. Infections that are acquired by patients or staff via a healthcare setting. Includes patient-to-staff transmission, staff-to-patient transmission and patient-to-patient transmission. Nosocomial transmission of influenza by these three means is well recognized.

Pandemic. When a novel influenza A virus spreads worldwide it is termed a pandemic (from the Greek *pan* meaning 'all' and *demos* meaning 'people').

Peak illness rate. The maximum rate (usually expressed as a percentage) of the population who will be ill at the same time during an influenza pandemic.

Personal protective measures. Infection control measures that individual people can undertake, e.g. hand washing and respiratory hygiene (see below).

Pre-pandemic vaccine. Vaccine produced in advance of a pandemic, containing antigens against a novel virus considered likely to cause a pandemic. The vaccine is procured in advance and might also be given in advance based on the likelihood that it may confer some protection against the actual pandemic virus. Note that an A/H5N1 pre-pandemic vaccine would not offer any protection against a pandemic caused by a different subtype, such as A/H1N1.

Priming. Exposure of naive immune cells to a specific antigen (e.g. the influenza A/H5N1 virus) enables them to differentiate into immune response cells (e.g. antibodies) or memory cells allowing a more rapid response upon re-exposure.

Prophylaxis. An intervention designed to prevent, rather than cure or treat a disease, that can be given either 'post' exposure (i.e. after exposure to the pathogen) or 'pre' exposure (i.e. in advance of exposure). The term is most commonly applied to the use of neuraminidase inhibitors for prophylaxis. Unlike vaccination, prophylaxis with antiviral drugs only lasts for as long as the medicine is taken.

Protective sequestration. A term used to describe when healthy people attempt to isolate themselves to reduce the risk of exposure to an infection. Rarely practical in relation to pandemic influenza, and leaves the individual susceptible unless vaccinated in the intervening period.

Public health countermeasures. Group actions taken that are intended to reduce human-to-human transmission of influenza and thereby mitigate the adverse effects of an epidemic or pandemic.

Quarantine. Applies to people exposed who may or may not be infected but are not ill. Separation or restriction of movement is then practised or applied in order that if any of these people subsequently become ill they will not pose a risk of infection to others.

Randomized controlled trial. A type of experiment used to test the efficacy of an intervention or medicine, which randomly allocates different interventions or medicines to the subjects in the trial, thereby reducing the chances of a biased result.

Real-time modelling. Real-time modelling, or 'nowcasting', is short-range forecasting based on current events to understand the evolving situation.

Reproductive number (R_0). Epidemiological term that describes the average number of people that one person with infection infects. If $R_0 > 1$, the number of infected people increases over time and transmission is sustained; if $R_0 < 1$ transmission is not sustained. The underlying R_0 of a pandemic virus affects the effectiveness of interventions and countermeasures.

Respirators. Face pieces that often have the external appearance of a simple 'mask' but are in fact specialist filtering devices that prevent the ingress of very small particles, e.g. infectious organisms, transmitted in aerosols.

Respiratory hygiene. Use of tissues to cover mouth and nostrils when coughing and sneezing and their correct disposal, followed by hand washing.

Secondary effects. The costs, risks and consequences of applying public health countermeasures and other interventions.

Self-isolation. Applies to people experiencing symptoms of influenza restricting their movements (in most cases, staying at home) and reducing their level of contact with other people (until symptom-free) in order to reduce the likelihood of onward transmission.

Social distancing. An imprecise term often applied to the collection of measures intended to decrease the frequency of contact among people and so possibly reduce influenza transmission. Most experts consider it better to describe the range of specific interventions within this blanket term.

Surgical masks. Masks worn when undertaking surgical procedures, mostly intended to prevent droplet transmission of respiratory infections from the wearer (not able to protect against aerosol transmission).

Zoonosis. When a disease is passed from an animal to man, it is called a zoonosis (from the Greek *zoon* meaning 'animal' and *nosos* meaning 'ill').

1 Seasonal Influenza: Epidemiology, Clinical Features and Surveillance

J. Van-Tam

- What is the public health importance of seasonal influenza?
- Is seasonal influenza related to pandemic influenza?
- What are the typical clinical features of influenza?
- Which age groups are most affected by seasonal influenza?
- Which groups are at highest risk?

1.1 Pandemic and Seasonal Influenza are Related Diseases

Developing a thorough understanding of pandemic influenza hinges upon first having a sound grasp of influenza as an 'everyday' illness. Influenza pandemics are relatively rare events compared with seasonal influenza, which inflicts human illness on a frequent basis. Furthermore, many inappropriate comparisons are drawn between pandemic influenza and avian influenza, especially when in reality a pandemic is more likely to resemble seasonal influenza than avian influenza. Indeed, pandemic and seasonal influenza are not separate entities; they represent a continuum of disease, from the emergence of a novel subtype in man (a pandemic) to the continued circulation of closely related viruses (of the same subtype) in subsequent years (seasonal influenza), sometimes several decades. For example, the A/H1N1 viruses that circulated from 1920 to 1956 were, in virological terms, descendants of the A/H1N1 virus, which emerged in 1918 and caused the 'Spanish influenza' pandemic (see Chapter 4), however, the epidemiology changed markedly over this period as the virus evolved (lost virulence) and population immunity increased. A closer look at the incidence of seasonal influenza shows that in the years immediately following a pandemic, subsequent epidemics tend to be relatively severe compared with those that occur several decades later. Figure 1.1 illustrates the incidence of influenza-like illness (ILI) from 1966 to 2007 in English general practices; the epidemics in the 1970s soon after the 'Hong Kong' pandemic wave in 1969–1970 are notably more severe than those in subsequent decades, although 1989–1990 was an outlier that may have been partially due to simultaneous respiratory syncytial virus (RSV) activity. Although seasonal influenza epidemics produce lower-level activity than pandemics, their repetitive annual nature means that cumulative morbidity and mortality probably exceed those associated with pandemic influenza. Consequently, seasonal influenza should not be underestimated as a major public health issue in its own right.

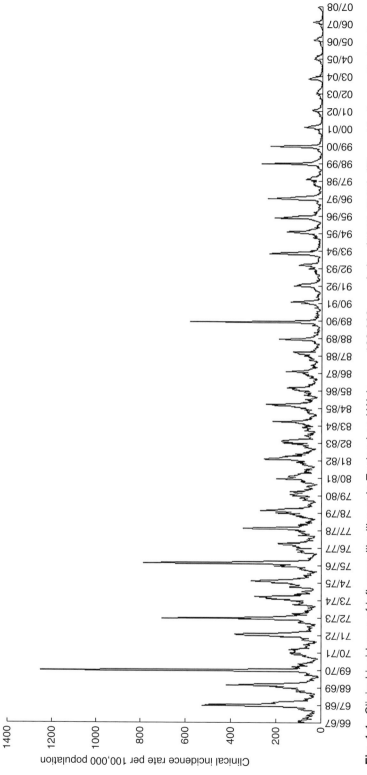

Fig. 1.1. Clinical incidence of influenza-like illness in England and Wales per 100,000 population (1967–2007). (Figure kindly supplied by the Royal College of General Practitioners' sentinel primary care network – Weekly Returns Service.)

J. Van-Tam

1.2   Influenza A and B

Although influenza virus has been categorized into three types, A, B and C, influenza C is but one of several hundred viruses that together account for the 'common cold' and is not considered further in this book. Influenza A and B are considered to be the major human pathogens responsible for seasonal influenza. They are clinically indistinguishable, although influenza B attack rates tend to be far higher in children than in adults. This is undoubtedly related to the inherent antigenic stability of influenza B compared with A, and the likelihood that exposure in childhood will generate longer cross-protective immunity (see Chapter 2). Nevertheless, re-infection with both influenza A and B is well recognized.

1.3   Clinical Features

Influenza in man presents as an acute illness characterized predominantly by cough, malaise and feverishness, typically of rapid onset. Other common additional symptoms are chills, headache, anorexia, coryza, myalgia and sore throat, which occur in 50 to 79% of confirmed cases; sputum, dizziness, hoarseness and chest pain in <50% of cases; vomiting and diarrhoea are also described but occur in <10% of cases. These features are quite non-specific, making it difficult to distinguish individual cases of influenza from other respiratory virus infections unless supported by surveillance data indicating the presence of influenza in the community. A typical illness lasts up to 5 days. In the vast majority of normal healthy individuals, influenza is self-limiting; however, even in these groups occasional severe illness is described, resulting rarely in unexpected death.

The biggest impact of seasonal influenza is felt through a range of associated secondary complications including acute bronchitis, pneumonia, otitis media (in children), myocarditis, pericarditis and neurological sequelae (febrile convulsions and Reye's syndrome in children; encephalitis in adults). The most common complication is acute bronchitis, but by far the most significant is bacterial pneumonia, where the common organisms described are *Streptococcus pneumoniae*, *Staphylococcus aureus* and *Haemophilus influenzae*. One of the least well-known facts about seasonal influenza is its strong association with electrocardiogram abnormalities, even in healthy adults, which frequently go unrecognized. Recovery from influenza may be followed by a period of fatigue and lethargy lasting several weeks.

Influenza is associated with more severe illness and higher rates of death and hospitalization in neonates and children under 2 years of age, pregnant women, the elderly (especially those over 75 years of age) and people with underlying co-morbidities (e.g. asthma, diabetes, chronic obstructive pulmonary disease (COPD), cardiac failure) in whom the acute infection may destabilize the underlying illness. With regard to possible differences between pandemic and seasonal influenza, it is not possible to predict in advance the clinical severity of the former compared with the latter, as the different pandemics of the 20th century produced greatly contrasting disease severity (see Chapter 4). Nevertheless, it is reasonable to surmise that a novel virus against which the population has little or no immunity on balance might be expected to produce an illness of longer duration, associated with prolonged virus excretion (see Chapter 5), compared with seasonal influenza.

1.4 Timing and Seasonality

The epidemiology of seasonal influenza is characterized in temperate zones of both the northern and southern hemispheres by epidemics of variable size that occur during the colder winter months, each one typically lasting 8–10 weeks. It is however important to note that influenza also occurs in tropical and subtropical zones; in these geographical areas where heat and humidity are year-round phenomena, there is an association of influenza activity with rainy seasons. Thus influenza in the tropics is not strictly seasonal (in the winter/summer sense) and may occur twice yearly in association with rainy periods. In the temperate zones where influenza activity is concentrated into the colder winter months, various theories have been advanced to explain this pattern, including: improved virus survival in conditions of low temperature and low humidity; low levels of ultraviolet radiation; and close congregation of people in domestic dwellings with low ventilation (windows closed). This concentration of disease activity makes epidemics rather more recognizable in temperate zones than in the tropics, because more acute pressure is generated on the healthcare system in a shorter period of time.

Usually one influenza A subtype (currently A/H3N2 or A/H1N1) or influenza B will dominate during a winter season, but this is far from always the case and 'mixed epidemics' are possible. In the northern hemisphere the timing of influenza B activity tends to be later in the season (generally after Christmas) than influenza A, but this is not a fixed rule. Unlike other infections such as RSV, the timing of onset varies markedly from season to season. Influenza activity is documented year-round (at low levels in summer) as are influenza outbreaks 'out of season', suggesting that virus circulates constantly.

While seasonal influenza is recognized to be seasonal in the temperate zones, traditionally pandemic influenza has not been regarded as seasonal to the same extent. For example, the first wave of the 1918 pandemic began in March 1918, in early spring. In the northern hemisphere, this wave was relatively small in size and mild in its clinical impact compared with the second wave in September 1918. It has since been suggested that the reason for the increased size and severity of the second wave might relate in part to seasonality, the timing of the resurgence in activity being influenced by the onset of autumn/winter conditions. Likewise, the 'Hong Kong' pandemic virus of 1968 did not appear in the UK until January 1969 and the main pandemic wave was then observed in the UK in the following winter season of 1969–1970 (Fig. 1.1); in contrast, the new virus entered the USA in early autumn 1968 and produced a large pandemic wave in the same winter of 1968–1969. If this observation is genuine, then if a future pandemic were to begin in the spring, more time might be gained for preparation and vaccine production, compared with the case of a novel virus appearing in early autumn at the start of the winter.

1.5 Burden of Illness and Clinical Attack Rates

In terms of its public health impact, seasonal influenza is often recognized as a disease of the elderly, the very young, and people with high-risk chronic illnesses such as COPD and diabetes. While this is true in one sense, in relation to the likelihood of death and hospitalization, from another perspective it is totally incorrect. Large

Table 1.1. Summary of age-specific influenza A serological attack rates observed in major community studies in the USA (Seattle, Washington; Tecumseh, Michigan; and Houston, Texas) during the 1970s.

Age group (years)	Attack rate (%)
<1	20–30
1–9	15–45
10–19	17–40
20–29	16–21
30–39	17–21
≥40	12–20

cohort studies of respiratory virus infection in families, which took place in the late 1960s and 1970s in the USA (Seattle, Washington; Tecumseh, Michigan; and Houston, Texas), have established that the highest annual attack rates for influenza occur in children and teenagers, and that these decline substantially with age; this is especially true for influenza B, which affects adults far less frequently. Typical values for serological attack rates described in the major cohort studies of the 1960s and 1970s are shown in Table 1.1. Roughly half were associated with symptomatic illness. The variability in attack rates reflects different populations, different seasons and different laboratory tests used between studies.

Of course, while attack rates in the young are highest, infection generally carries fewer consequences in children over 2 years old, teenagers and healthy adults, with correspondingly low levels of morbidity, mortality and hospitalization. Thus, seasonal influenza is somewhat paradoxical with the highest attack rates in the young but the greatest public health impact in the elderly. It is especially noteworthy that about 50% of influenza infections (as confirmed by serology) appear to be asymptomatic. This contradicts the popular myth that genuine influenza is always associated with prostration and debility, and that anything less severe could only be 'just a cold'. In fact, interesting data from healthcare workers in Glasgow, Scotland during an influenza A epidemic in 1993–1994 revealed that, of 518 workers (mainly nursing staff), 23% showed evidence of infection (based on serological findings) by the end of the season. However, 28% of those who had seroconverted could not recall any kind of respiratory illness that winter, and 52% had not taken time off work. Thus clear opportunities for transmission within the hospital environment were revealed.

1.6 Influenza in Children

Until fairly recently, the impact of influenza in young children (aged less than 2 years) had been poorly appreciated; however, it is now clear that the level of influenza-related hospitalizations in this age group is as high as in adults with high-risk under-lying conditions. Children represent a special epidemiological phenomenon in relation to influenza, because they have poor respiratory etiquette and are known to excrete virus for longer and in higher titres than their adult counterparts. The risk of acquisition of influenza among adults is raised within households containing young children and there are epidemiological data which clearly indicate that during influenza epidemics, school sickness absence and paediatric admissions peak 1 to 2 weeks earlier than workplace absenteeism and hospital admissions in adults within the same community. These data strongly suggest that children act as sentinels for influenza activity within communities and play a major role in propagating transmission in households and communities. These points are highly relevant in relation to infection control practices and possible pandemic countermeasures such as school closures (see Chapter 10) and vaccination (see Chapter 9).

1.7 Diagnostic Certainty

One of the biggest problems related to fully estimating the burden of seasonal influenza relates to case ascertainment. Until the advent of neuraminidase inhibitors (see Chapter 8), there were few realistic or practical options for the treatment of influenza and thus no clear advantages in confirming the diagnosis using virological tests. Even with the availability of neuraminidase inhibitors, the cost, complexity and timeliness of diagnostic tests make it neither practical nor economical to confirm the illness before commencing treatment; instead therapy should generally be initiated on clinical suspicion and information from surveillance data. Influenza-related hospitalization frequently occurs due to disease complications; there is again little perceived clinical value in making a diagnosis of influenza at this late stage in the illness and indeed less chance of a positive test several days after the onset of symptoms. Thus, in all probability, true disease burden remains significantly underestimated.

1.8 Excess Mortality

Despite the lack of established culture within healthcare systems for making a definitive diagnosis of influenza, severe epidemics have always achieved prominence through societal disruption and a phenomenon known as excess mortality; in essence, a large number of unexpected deaths brought together in time and space by the occurrence of influenza – the ultimate example being pandemic influenza itself. This phenomenon was first noted by historical writers (usually ecclesiastical) who chronicled outbreaks of 'epidemic fevers' stretching back several centuries (see Chapter 4), some of which will have been due to influenza. Modern epidemiological techniques have now been applied to the same basic observations in order to quantify the number of 'excess deaths' during a period of known influenza activity. Provided the source data are robust, this calculation can be performed retrospectively or prospectively. All methodologies are based around the calculation of a relevant 'baseline' for deaths (allowing for seasonal variations) and then calculating the surplus of deaths over and above that baseline that coincide with periods of known influenza activity. One of the main findings during influenza epidemics is that deaths which are actually ascribed to influenza during death certification represent a relatively small proportion (about 10%) of the total excess deaths observed. The remainder are ascribed to secondary complications (e.g. pneumonia) and underlying chronic illnesses (e.g. cardiac failure). Thus, it is now accepted convention that

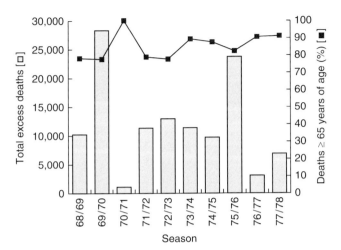

Fig. 1.2. Estimated excess deaths among adults attributable to influenza and the percentage in people aged ≥65 years, England and Wales (1968–69 to 1977–78 winter seasons). (Data from Tillet *et al.*, 1983; reproduced from an original by J.S. Nguyen-Van-Tam; first appeared in Nguyen-Van-Tam, J.S. (1998) Epidemiology of Influenza. In: Nicholson, K.G., Webster, R.G. and Hay, A.J. (eds) *Textbook of Influenza*. Blackwell Science, Oxford.)

all-cause mortality should be considered when estimating the burden of mortality associated with influenza.

It is now clear that influenza epidemics frequently produce excess mortality, which is mainly seen in the elderly. On occasions, the excess deaths noted during an epidemic are followed by a much smaller deficit in deaths over the next few weeks, suggesting that influenza kills some frail and elderly people whose deaths would have occurred soon in any case; while probably true, these still represent a minority of all excess deaths. During the last large influenza epidemic in the UK in 1989–1990 it is estimated that 29,000 excess deaths occurred in a period of about 60 days, almost entirely in people aged 75 years and over. Even after adjusting for a post-epidemic deficit, the excess death toll was still about 17,000. It is estimated that there were about 36,000 influenza-related deaths per annum in the USA during the relatively mild decade, 1990–1999. Excess deaths due to influenza do not occur to the same extent every season, indeed they are highly variable, however, one remarkable consistency is in their age distribution. At least 80% of seasonal influenza excess deaths occur in individuals aged 65 and over (Fig. 1.2). Of course this may not be the case during a pandemic, and potential changes in the pattern of age-specific mortality are discussed in Chapter 4.

1.9 High-risk Illnesses

The risk of seasonal influenza-related complications, hospitalization and death rises with age; the first noticeable impact can be seen from the age of 50 years but rates continue to rise sharply after this. In relation to hospital admissions, the extent of the problem in public health terms is disproportionately felt beyond 75 years of age, because lengths of hospital stay increase markedly at this point. Thus age on its own can be regarded as a major risk factor for complications and deaths due to seasonal influenza.

However, in addition to age per se, it is also well recognized that the rates of secondary complications, hospitalizations and deaths due to seasonal influenza infection are higher in individuals with certain underlying co-morbidities, compared with those who are healthy. Not only do these patients appear more vulnerable to influenza, the infection can also destabilize or decompensate underlying conditions such as diabetes, angina and cardiac failure. Similar observations have been made from multiple epidemiological studies and there is very solid agreement that 'high-risk' groups can be defined as those with chronic respiratory disease (asthma, COPD), chronic heart disease, diabetes, renal disease, significant immunosupression and pregnant women. In turn, this explains the remarkable international consistency regarding the core groups recommended for annual influenza vaccination. The clear observation that individuals who are immune-suppressed are at greater risk from seasonal influenza clearly raises significant public health concerns about the potential impact of a novel, virulent pandemic virus in parts of the world affected by a high prevalence of HIV, most notably sub-Saharan Africa and parts of Asia. Although not a high-risk illness, smoking has also been identified as a relevant risk factor. In the Israeli military, clinical attack rates during an epidemic were higher in the same unit among smokers than non-smokers, and other studies suggest that illness severity and sickness absence due to influenza are increased in smokers compared with non-smokers.

The identification of high-risk groups has driven annual demand for seasonal influenza vaccines around the world; in turn, this drives not only the availability of manufacturing capacity for a future pandemic vaccine, but also policy assumptions about the size and composition of high-risk groups that might be targeted for specific pandemic interventions. Given the fact that unexpected subgroups of the population proved to be at high risk during the 1918 pandemic (young adults), and might be so again in the future, this is a difficult area of policy setting that illustrates the need for effective real-time surveillance during a pandemic.

1.10 Nosocomial Infection and Outbreaks in Semi-closed Communities

Outbreaks in hospitals, nursing homes and boarding schools are a notable and common feature of seasonal influenza. In a review of 41 nursing homes outbreaks in the USA, an average attack rate among residents of 43% was recorded during epidemic periods and 16% at other times. Attack rates in boarding school outbreaks appear highly variable, ranging from 20 to 90% in the published literature. These most often occur during periods of known community influenza activity but are also well-described 'out-of-season', before and after periods of wider community activity. In general, they can be successfully interrupted by the application of cohorted care and strict droplet and contact precautions (see Chapter 5). Outbreaks that occur prior to the onset of widespread seasonal activity often do so in boarding schools, which can act as sentinel institutions, giving early warning of more widespread community activity. Outbreaks that occur in nursing homes towards the end of the winter season have been attributed to drifted strains against which the annual vaccine (given some 6 months previously) is no longer a close match. Likewise, even when vaccine and wild viruses are considered to be still well-matched at the end of the season, waning of antibodies in elderly vaccinees has been attributed as the cause of outbreaks. Risk factors for influenza outbreaks in closed institutions include: low influenza vaccine uptake; a large number of residents living in close proximity to each other; and allowing staff members to be employed part-time in other institutions (potential for nosocomial spread between sites). In long-term care establishments, there are persuasive data that suggest that vaccination of staff reduces mortality among residents (irrespective of the latter's vaccination status); yet influenza vaccine uptake among health and social care workers generally remains low. Mortality rates tend to be highest in institutions housing the frail elderly and the immune-suppressed; for example, mortality rates of up to 70% have been described due to influenza outbreaks in stem cell transplant units. These types of institutions will present critical infection control issues in the event of a future pandemic.

1.11 Surveillance Data on Seasonal Influenza and Pandemic Needs

Data that define the timing of influenza activity and quantify its impact are needed for both seasonal and pandemic influenza. Table 1.2 summarizes the types of surveillance data currently available for seasonal influenza, and their advantages and limitations.

Influenza surveillance remains rudimentary in many parts of the world. This leaves potentially large gaps and areas of near 'blackout' in relation to the early detection of human respiratory disease that might offer the only chance of an early warning of the next pandemic (or some other novel respiratory pathogen; e.g. severe acute respiratory syndrome, SARS). One of the best coordinated regions of the world is Europe, characterized by the surveillance systems within the EISN (European Influenza Surveillance Network).

During an influenza pandemic, the surveillance systems that are currently deployed for seasonal influenza will need to be continued. However, there will be a much greater emphasis on obtaining the data in real time because 'nowcasting' (see Chapter 7), assessment of pandemic severity (Chapter 10) and the timing of public health and pharmaceutical countermeasures will all depend upon gaining a rapid understanding of the epidemiological features of the emerging crisis. However, certain data sources will potentially be less useful and have drawbacks. For example, sentinel primary care data will strongly underestimate the incidence of pandemic illness if the designated route of access to antiviral medication is designed specifically to avoid primary care; once hospital capacity is saturated at the peak of a pandemic, admissions data will not reflect demand for hospital-level care. New surveillance systems may be needed to supplement existing ones. These cannot be easily invented or introduced when a pandemic starts, instead they need to be designed, piloted and validated in advance. Such systems are under development in some countries, for example, the UK plans to use a dedicated information collection system to gather early-stage epidemiological data on the pandemic, and to have a separate clinical information network to gather data relevant to the clinical management of pandemic influenza throughout the pandemic period.

Table 1.2. Seasonal influenza surveillance sources: main advantages, limitations and issues especially relevant to pandemic deployment (**P**).

Source	Advantages	Limitations
Sentinel primary care data	Estimates clinical incidence if linked to known population Can be linked to virology data to corroborate clinical diagnosis and to vaccination records to estimate vaccine effectiveness Provides age-specific data	Based on clinical diagnosis of ILI, with or without formal case definition Cannot record ILI cases that do not consult with primary care practitioner (those 'below the radar screen') (**P**) May offer skewed data in a pandemic if cases are re-routed to deliberately bypass primary care
Sickness absence data (including schools)	Can be obtained within the workplace or school, or from statutory sickness benefit claims Can be related to periods of known influenza activity (**P**) May help to identify economic cost of lost productivity and wider societal impact Boarding school data may give early warning of increase in community activity	Cause of absence not always stated Scope for significant misdiagnosis if self-certified data are used (**P**) School data disrupted during holiday periods and possible pandemic closures (**P**) During a pandemic, workplace absence may be due to illness, third-party leave (caring for children) or fear of attending work
Hospital admissions data	Can be related to periods of known influenza activity Useful to quantify excess healthcare demand Can be broken down by cause of admission (e.g. cardiac, respiratory) (**P**) Can provide clinical data on process of care, prognosis, dependency, case fatality, etc.	(**P**) Difficult to obtain in real time, except basic raw numbers Relevant acute admissions need to be separated from others (elective, non-influenza) (**P**) Once hospital system saturated will not be able to measure further (unmet) need for hospital care
Laboratory virology data	Highly accurate influenza-specific data confirm definite community activity Data available by subtype and strain (**P**) Testing for antiviral drug resistance is possible May be linked to clinical data in some schemes (**P**) Provides data on other respiratory virus pathogens mistaken for influenza	Specimens not usually taken from all patients – significant sampling bias unless sampling protocol overrides Estimation of incidence not possible Data yield highly dependent on quality of both clinical specimens and receiving laboratory Serological data difficult to obtain, especially convalescent serum

Data source	Advantages	Limitations
Sales of over-the-counter cough/cold/flu remedies	(P) Captures data on cases who do not visit general practitioner	Highly non-specific May be commercial-in-confidence, therefore unavailable in many settings Fails to capture those who medicate with simple antipyretics (paracetamol) or who take nothing (P) Sales data could reflect advanced stocking up early in the pandemic
Calls to sickness helplines and Internet search counts	Spreads net wider than primary care consultations and pharmacy purchases (P) If helpline linked to antiviral treatment allocation, may estimate true population incidence	Biased towards patients who actively seek advice Based on self-diagnosis and patient reporting of symptoms Significant 'background noise'
Mortality data	Gives view of societal impact Determines most susceptible groups (e.g. young adults in 1918) Calculation of excess mortality is possible	(P) In some systems, considerable delay between date of death and recording in official statistics Only small proportion of total influenza-related deaths ascribed to influenza as the primary cause of death (P) Shortage of physicians and large number of simultaneous deaths may further reduce accurate certification during a pandemic

ILI, influenza-like illness.

1.12 Summary

A great deal is known about the epidemiology of 'seasonal influenza'; this provides essential background knowledge for an understanding of pandemic influenza. Seasonal influenza is characterized by periods of activity lasting 8 to 10 weeks that are unpredictable in their precise timing although clearly seasonal in the temperate zones. Morbidity and mortality are concentrated at the extremes of age, notably children under 2 years of age and the elderly; however, people of any age with certain chronic illnesses are also more severely affected. Excess mortality varies from year to year but is generally concentrated in the elderly. Annual vaccination is recommended for those at increased risk of complications and death; in most countries with active policies, this entails targeted vaccination of people aged 65 and over, adults with high-risk conditions, health and social care workers, and sometimes young children.

Understanding the epidemiology of seasonal influenza teaches the pandemic planner the general principles of how influenza behaves in human populations and how this can be monitored. Similar data on the epidemiology of an emerging pandemic virus will be needed within a rapid timeframe in order to inform forecasting, severity assessment and the deployment of countermeasures.

1.13 Summary Points

- Seasonal influenza is of major public health importance. Epidemics cause disruption and excess morbidity and mortality.
- Seasonal influenza viruses are virological descendants of previous pandemic viruses.
- Seasonal influenza is difficult to distinguish from other respiratory virus infections that circulate simultaneously each winter in the northern and southern hemispheres. The most significant features are cough, feverishness and rapid onset, but a large range of other symptoms is also possible.
- Seasonal influenza is a disease characterized by high attack rates in young children and teenagers, but the biggest effect on morbidity and mortality is in the elderly.
- The elderly and individuals with 'high-risk' underlying illnesses are at greatest risk from influenza and should be targeted for annual vaccination.

Further Reading

Elder, A.G., O'Donnell, B., McCruden, E.A.B., Symington, I.S. and Carman, W.F. (1996) Incidence and recall of influenza in a cohort of Glasgow healthcare workers during the 1993–94 epidemic: results of serum testing and questionnaire. *British Medical Journal* 313, 1241–1242.

Fleming, D.M. and Elliot, A.J. (2008) Lessons from 40 years' surveillance of influenza in England and Wales. *Epidemiology and Infection* 136, 866–875.

Fox, J.P., Cooney, M.K., Hall, C.E. and, Foy, M.F. (1982) Influenza virus infections in Seattle families, 1975–79. II. Pattern of infection in invaded households and relation of age and prior antibody to occurrence of infection and related illness. *American Journal of Epidemiology* 116, 228–242.

Glezen, W.P. and Couch, R.B. (1978) Interpandemic influenza in the Houston area, 1974–76. *New England Journal of Medicine* 298, 587–592.

Hall, C.E., Cooney, M.K. and Fox, J.P. (1973) The Seattle Virus Watch: IV. Comparative epidemiologic observations of infections with influenza A and B viruses, 1965–69, in families with young children. *American Journal of Epidemiology* 98, 365–380.

Monto, A.S. and Kiouhmehr, F. (1975) The Tecumseh study of respiratory illness. IX. Occurrence of influenza in the community, 1966–1971. *American Journal of Epidemiology* 102, 553–563.

Nguyen-Van-Tam, J.S. (1998) Epidemiology of influenza. In: Nicholson, K.G., Webster, R.G. and Hay, A.J. (eds) *Textbook of Influenza*. Blackwell Science Ltd, Oxford, UK, pp. 181–206.

Teo, S.S., Nguyen-Van-Tam, J.S. and Booy, R. (2005) Influenza burden of illness, diagnosis, treatment and prevention: what is the evidence in children and where are the gaps? *Archives of Disease in Childhood* 90, 532–536.

Tillett, H.E., Smith, J.W.G. and Gooch, C.D. (1983) Excess deaths attributable to influenza in England and Wales: age at deaths and certified cause. *International Journal of Epidemiology* 12, 344–352.

World Health Organization (2009) *Epidemic and Pandemic Alert and Response (EPR). Global surveillance during an influenza pandemic*. Version 1 (updated draft April 2009). http://www.who.int/csr/resources/publications/swineflu/surveillance/en/index.html (accessed June 2009).

2 Basic Influenza Virology and Immunology

L.R. HAAHEIM

- How do antibodies against haemagglutinin and neuraminidase differ in the way they interfere with the viral replication cycle?
- How do amantadine, rimantadine and the neuraminidase-inhibitor drugs work?
- What role does cell-mediated immunity play in combating influenza infection?
- What is immunological memory?
- What is meant by 'priming' a population with for example a pre-pandemic vaccine?

2.1 Introduction

Influenza virology and immunology are immensely complex subjects. Nevertheless, the non-specialist requires a certain understanding of both in order to understand the origins of past influenza pandemics (Chapter 4), the threat posed by novel influenza viruses (Chapter 3) and the role of possible countermeasures such as vaccines (Chapter 9) and antiviral drugs (Chapter 8). It is important to understand that all viruses are intracellular obligate parasites. This is just another way of saying that the virus cannot replicate unless it gets inside a host cell. Briefly, a virus is a piece of genetic material, protected by proteins and in some cases also by a membrane, on the look-out for a cell to invade so that it can re-programme the cell to make copies of itself (the virus).

2.2 The Virus

Despite the abundance of exotic names given to influenza viruses and their somewhat mystical and confusing nomenclature, there are in fact only three types of influenza virus: type A, B and C, the former of which can be divided into a range of subtypes. They all belong to the *Orthomyxoviridae* family of viruses (from the Greek *myxa* meaning 'mucus'). As influenza viruses are changing slightly and gradually over time, there is also a range of strains (also known as 'variants' or 'isolates') to consider. Type B is mainly a human pathogen and causes occasional winter outbreaks and epidemics, whereas type C gives only mild or unapparent disease and is considered to be one of the several hundred viruses that together cause the syndrome known as the 'common cold'. However, this chapter focuses on influenza type A, which is the only type of influenza associated with pandemic influenza.

©CAB International 2010. *Introduction to Pandemic Influenza* (eds J.S. Nguyen-Van-Tam and C. Sellwood)

The influenza virus is a medium-sized enveloped virus with a segmented negative-sense RNA as its nucleic acid. This means that the viral RNA (vRNA) cannot function as a messenger RNA (mRNA) to translate the genetic information to viral proteins. The influenza genome has eight separate segments coding for ten different proteins, of which eight are structural (Table 2.1 and Fig. 2.1).

By electron microscopy one can visualize spikes on the viral surface; these are the surface proteins haemagglutinin (HA) and neuraminidase (NA). Sometimes one can discern the internal components as bundles of segmented striped filaments. These are the nucleoproteins surrounding the viral RNA (Fig. 2.2).

Influenza A is the most important of the three influenza types; it is found in a range of animal species (e.g. birds, pigs, horses, minks, seals, whales; Table 2.2) and has the capacity to cause pandemics. The type A influenza is divided into several subtypes based on the properties of the surface proteins HA and NA.

Birds, and particularly aquatic birds, form the natural animal reservoir for all known influenza A subtypes. In most cases influenza in birds is a benign or unapparent intestinal infection. The current list of 16 HA subtypes and nine NA subtypes may well expand with time. This vast pool of influenza genes represents a potential contagious threat to man, as there are currently only some varying degrees of pre-existing immunity to the H1, H2 and H3 haemagglutinins and to the N1 and N2 neuraminidases. On rare occasions, novel viruses may cross the species barrier and infect people (see Chapter 3).

Table 2.1. Gene segments of influenza A virus, in decreasing size order.

Segment	Name	Function
1	PB2	Polymerase complex. Viral replication
2	PB1(-F2)	
3	PA	
4	HA	Haemagglutinin, a glycosylated surface protein. Initiates infection by binding to cellular receptors. Antigenically highly variable, 16 subtypes
5	NP	Nucleoprotein, encapsidates the RNA segments. The RNA–NP complex is designated RNP
6	NA	Neuraminidase, a glycosylated surface protein. Enzyme that splits off newly made virus from host cell. Antigenically variable, nine subtypes. Blocked by the new anti-neuraminidase drugs[a]
7	M1	Matrix protein. Located under the surface lipid layer. Antigenically very stable, but type-specific (A, B, C)
	M2	Ion channel, just a few copies in the viral membrane. Antigenically very stable. Blocked by the adamantane drugs[b]
8	NS1 NS2 (NEP)	Non-structural proteins, functions not well understood. NS1 is assumed to inhibit the host's interferon synthesis. NS2 helps in exporting the viral RNA complexed with NP to the cytoplasm

[a]Oseltamivir and zanamivir.
[b]Amantadine and rimantadine.

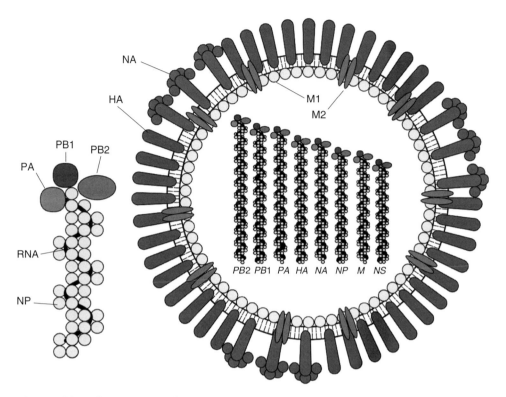

Fig. 2.1. The influenza virus. (Courtesy of KarlAlbert Brokstad, University of Bergen.)

Table 2.2. Distribution of influenza A subtypes among some animal species.[a,b,c,d]

HA subtype	Found in	NA subtype	Found in
H1	Man, swine, birds	N1	Man, swine, birds
H2	Man, birds	N2	Man, swine, birds
H3	Man, swine, horse, birds	N3	Birds
H4	Birds	N4	Birds
H5	Birds	N5	Birds
H6	Birds	N6	Birds
H7	Horse, birds	N7	Horse, birds
H8	Birds	N8	Horse, birds
H9	Birds	N9	Birds
H10	Birds		
H11	Birds		
H12	Birds		
H13	Birds		
H14	Birds		
H15	Birds		
H16	Birds		

[a]Avian A/H5, A/H7 and A/H9 strains have sporadically infected man to give systemic disease.
[b]Fowl plague is caused by high-pathogenic variants of the subtypes A/H5 and A/H7.
[c]Strains of the A/H3N2 and A/H1N1 (and A/H1N2) subtypes circulate in human subjects today.
[d]The 'bird flu' from South-east Asia belongs to the A/H5N1 subtype.

L.R. Haaheim

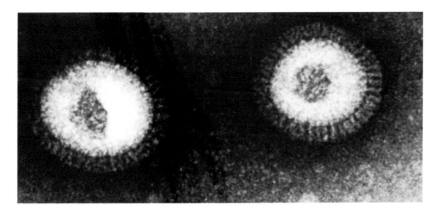

Fig. 2.2. Electron micrograph showing two virus particles, approximate diameter is 100–150 nm. The surface proteins haemagglutinin and neuraminidase can be seen as spikes, and the nucleoprotein can be seen through the damaged viral membrane. (Courtesy of WHO Collaborating Centre for Reference and Research on Influenza, Melbourne, Australia; micrographs prepared by Ross Hamilton.)

2.3 Nomenclature

The current system of nomenclature dates back to 1980 and designates the type/animal host/geographical place of isolation/strain number/year of isolation (two or four digits) and, if type A, followed by a bracket with H and N subtype designation. This system was initially based on antigenic differences and similarities between viruses, mostly based on the haemagglutination-inhibition test (see later). In recent years, advances in the rapid genetic characterization of viruses has enabled the construction of phylogenetic (family) trees that offer a much more detailed picture of the relationship between viruses. It is in this context that the term 'clade' is used to cluster genetically related strains into smaller groups.

For influenza viruses isolated from animals, the species in question is listed, for example:

- A/swine/Iowa/15/1930 (H1N1) (in earlier literature the H1 in this case was designated Hsw1).
- A/equine/Miami/1/1963 (H3N8).
- A/gull/Maryland/704/1977 (H13N6).
- A/seal/Massachusetts/1/1980 (H7N7).
- A/bar-headed goose/Quinghai/1A/2005 (H5N1).

In pre-1980 publications, H1 isolates made before 1946 were designated H0.

The human isolate A/Anhui/1/2005 (H5N1) was from a zoonotic case in 2005 where a person in Anhui Province, China was infected with an avian H5N1 strain. This style of nomenclature can become complicated, for example, in the case of A/turkey/Turkey/1/2005 (H5N1), a virus isolated from a turkey in Turkey in 2005.

Typically, the nomenclature of human influenza strains is most frequently encountered by the non-virologist in relation to the World Health Organization

(WHO) recommendations for seasonal influenza vaccine antigen composition; for example, for the northern hemisphere for 2009–2010:

- A/Brisbane/59/2007 (H1N1)-like virus.
- A/Brisbane/10/2007 (H3N2)-like virus.
- B/Brisbane/60/2008-like virus.

This is an extremely rare situation where all three recommended strains by chance happen to come from the same geographical location.

Important examples

A much-used classical human strain, the so-called PR8 virus, has the formulation A/Puerto Rico/8/34 (H1N1). The PR8 strain is a frequently used partner when high-yielding seed strains are prepared for vaccine purposes (see Chapter 9). The Spanish influenza virus is exemplified by the strain A/Brevig Mission/1/1918 (H1N1), the Asian influenza pandemic in 1957 by A/Singapore/1/1957 (H2N2), and the Hong Kong pandemic of 1968 by A/Hong Kong/1/1968 (H3N2).

2.4 Replication

Step 1: the virus hooks on to the host cells

The virus must find somewhere on the host cell surface to attach to and initiate the first step in a long and complicated process of making more identical copies of itself. Viruses are opportunistic agents, and make use of existing host cell features that have beneficial primary purposes other than serving as attachment points for pathogens. Different viruses (other than influenza) have different preferences for the cellular membrane structures they select to use as an anchor point.

The haemagglutinin spikes on the influenza virus attach to human cells at an N-acetylneuraminic acid (sialic acid) residue attached to a sugar molecule (N-glucosamine); these are abundant on the epithelial cells in human airways. The precise chemical bond between the sialic acid and the sugar molecule determines whether human influenza viruses or avian viruses can bind to the respiratory epithelial cells. Human influenza strains preferably bind to so-called α-2,6 linked receptors, whereas avian strains prefer an α-2,3 linkage. This distinction is not absolute. In man most of the receptors are of the α-2,6 type, but α-2,3 structures are apparently present in the lower airways.

Pigs, as an interesting case, have both types of receptors throughout their airways and are believed to be a likely mixing vessel allowing them to be doubly infected by human and avian viruses to generate new gene constellations. It is possible that the pandemics of 1957 and 1968 both arose because pigs served as a mixing vessel for an avian and a circulating human strain to generate a new human pandemic virus (Figs 2.3 and 2.4).

Pandemic mode 1

Pigs have receptors for both avian and human influenza viruses. A doubly infected pig may select a reassortant virus that could infect and spread among people (as probably happened in 1957 and 1968).

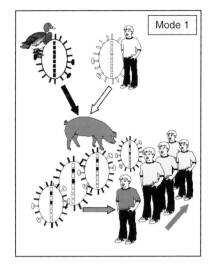

Pandemic mode 2

Man could be infected with an avian influenza virus. Through accumulations of point mutations (genetic adaptation) a variant could arise that could spread efficiently from person to person. This mode was probably the mechanism behind the appearance of the A/H1N1 Spanish influenza in 1918.

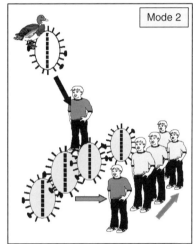

Pandemic mode 3

Man could simultaneously be infected with both avian and human influenza viruses. A reassortant virus could be selected that could infect and spread amomg people. So far not a documented pandemic mode, but human–human reassortants have been documented (currently A/H3N2 + A/H1N1 to give A/H1N2).

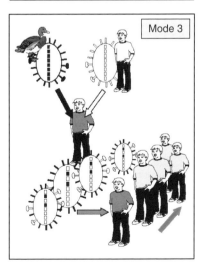

Fig. 2.3. Pandemic mode.

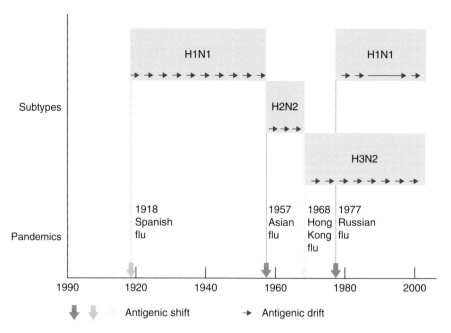

Fig. 2.4. Antigenic shifts and pandemics in the 20th century. (This image was first published in Wilschut, J.C., McElhaney, J.E. and Palache, A.M. (2006) *Influenza Rapid Reference*, 2nd Edition. Elsevier Ltd, p. 63.

Step 2: the virus enters the cell and starts replicating itself

The next and important step is to enter the cell. This is done by a process called receptor-mediated endocytosis, in which the cellular membrane invaginates and encloses the virus particle, thus creating an endosome (a vesicle) inside the cell. This in itself will not suffice, as the virus is still separated from the cell's machinery and will need to enter the cytoplasm. A two-step process does this. First, the endosome allows protons to enter, so creating an acid environment which produces a conformational change in the HA molecule, enabling it to fuse with the endosomal membrane. Simultaneously, protons are also pumped inside the virus particle itself, dissociating the M1 protein and the RNA–nucleoprotein complex (RNP), allowing the latter to enter the cytoplasm and migrate to the cell nucleus. It is a protein in the viral membrane designated M2 that performs this ion-channel function. The classical anti-influenza A drugs, amantadine and rimantadine, block the M2 activity and thus abort or slow down the replication process.

The subsequent steps in the replication cycle are many and rather complicated, but the viral nucleic acid migrates to the nucleus where two processes take place: one is to use the virus' own replicative enzymes to make copies of the incoming viral RNA, the other is to make a positive strand of the viral RNA that can function as messenger RNA for subsequent protein synthesis in the cytoplasm. The net effect is to take over the host cell and produce virus proteins and RNA.

Step 3: new viruses are released and ready to infect new cells

When the newly made proteins and genetic material have been produced, the viral surface proteins (HA, NA and M2) assemble on the cellular membrane and the other viral proteins locate themselves just under the now modified cellular membrane. Through a budding process, new virus-like spheres are ready to be set free. Each haemagglutinin spike on the viral surface is a trimer consisting of three identical HA proteins held together by non-covalent bonds. For an influenza virus particle to be infectious, the HA monomers must undergo cleavage by trypsin-like enzymes from the host organism. This is essential, as the influenza virus does not code for its own proteolytic enzymes. In most cases with human influenza strains, such enzymes are abundant in the respiratory airways, either secreted by certain epithelial cells or from resident bacteria. In highly pathogenic avian viruses the HA molecule is modified slightly, making it sensitive to cleavage by intracellular host enzymes in a range of tissues, thus allowing viral spread to multiple organs.

The final release of newly made virus is aided by the viral NA enzyme splitting off the sialic acid, which holds the HA of the new virus bound to the host cell. The NA here acts like a midwife facilitating the release of new viruses. This is the mechanism that is blocked by the new anti-influenza drugs – the neuraminidase inhibitors. These drugs do not stop the virus from infecting the cell, but rather interfere with the release of newly made viruses from cells already infected. Once the newly made virus is detached it will attempt to infect a new cell. The cycle continues, leaving in its wake dead epithelial cells, until the host's immune system stops it. But as long as new viruses are produced, the host may be contagious to others if the concentration of virus in sputum, nasal discharges or cough droplets is sufficient. Usually, an otherwise sound and healthy person will be contagious for 2–4 days after onset of clinical illness, usually when the patient is febrile. Importantly, there are some indications that an infected person may be contagious for a short period (1 day or so) before the onset of clinical illness, but this is not adequately known at the present time (see Chapter 5).

2.5 The Immune Response

The innate response

The innate response is the first line of defence, sometimes called 'natural immunity'. Having negotiated the physical barriers such as the mucus lining and cilia in the airways, the main defence players are a range of white blood cells such as the natural killer cells, macrophages and granulocytes in the invaded tissue, as well as a special set of cells called dendritic cells. The latter have long projections from their surfaces (dendrites) allowing efficient scanning and uptake of foreign material; they are particularly active in recognizing certain predefined structures from external sources (e.g. infectious agents). They and other cells, like macrophages and granulocytes, will take up, destroy and process the foreign material and initiate the adaptive immune system. They are therefore also called antigen-presenting cells (APCs). It is particularly important to know that the innate immune system has no ability to adapt to (i.e. learn from) its previous experience. The innate response is the first line of defence and is able to react immediately before the adaptive response is ready, which could take 3–4 days. Without the innate immune system, we would have serious problems combating even the most insignificant of infections.

The adaptive immune response

The humoral response

The B-lymphocytes have pre-formed antibodies on their surfaces acting like receptors for foreign material. After an intricate sequence of antigenic stimulation and re-shuffling of the gene complexes coding for the various parts of the immunoglobulin proteins, they end up as antibody-secreting cells, the final stage being the plasma cells secreting fine-tuned antibodies. These cells can be described as specialized factories secreting large quantities of antibodies that are tailor-made to the antigen in question. Not all antibodies are equally well adapted to bind to the antigen; they differ in affinity (binding strength) to the antigen. Some antibodies have the capacity to recognize a wider range of different antigenic structures; they are cross-reactive. Another arm of the B-cell activation process is to generate memory cells. They will home into and reside in the bone marrow. At random intervals they will leave and be on the look-out for recognizable antigenic material and, if this is found, be reactivated to form new plasma cells. As a bonus, new and fresh memory cells will be generated as well. Additionally, it is also recognized that the bone marrow may harbour certain long-lived plasma cells continuously secreting antibodies for years if not for life.

The cellular response

Although antibodies are particularly good at neutralizing free virus and recognizing viral proteins on infected cells, an equally significant arm of the immune response is the generation of helper and cytotoxic T-lymphocytes. The latter will find and destroy host cells exhibiting foreign material (e.g. fragments of viral structures) on their surface. T-cells, like B-cells, have specialized receptors on their surface able to recognize foreign material. A requirement for binding to a foreign structure of an infected cell is that the fragment is presented, or literally 'served', on a class 1 major histocompatibility complex (MHC) on the surface of the host cell, signalling that an infection is in progress. Most cells in our body have such MHC class 1 molecules. The antibody response, on the other hand, requires the assistance of T-helper cells. For these cells to recognize foreign material, the fragments must be presented on a class 2 histocompatibility complex. The MHC class 2 complex is found only on APCs such as macrophages, B-lymphocytes and dendritic cells. There is a large degree of cooperation between the initial innate response and between the two subsequent arms of the adaptive response, sending chemical messages (lymphokines and cytokines) between them to refine and direct the appropriate immune reaction.

2.6   The Variable Virus

Antigenic drift

Most RNA viruses have a poor proof-reading mechanism, leading to errors and mistakes during the replication cycles. The influenza viruses in particular seem to be promiscuous and to a large extent accept these 'mistakes' without compromising the required three-dimensional structures of the viral proteins, in particular the HA and NA on the viral surface. These subtle changes are called 'antigenic drift' and are minor differences in the antigenic make-up that may manifest themselves as new field variants ('strains', 'isolates') that could cause winter outbreaks and epidemics. For the human population previous immunological experience against viruses of previous seasons will to some extent protect an individual, at least against serious infections. At the same time, herd immunity in the population is likely to facilitate the emergence of new and antigenically 'drifted' strains. It is assumed that subclinical infections occur frequently. This should be considered as an advantage, as it may allow boosting and refreshing of pre-existing cross-reactive immunological memory. Such minor antigenic changes are seen almost every winter. It is therefore important for the efficacy of trivalent seasonal influenza vaccines that they keep abreast with the changing viruses in the field. This is the reason why the WHO updates its vaccine strain recommendation twice yearly, once per hemisphere.

Antigenic shift and reassortment

More fundamental changes are necessary for a pandemic to take place. This is designated 'antigenic shift' and is seen when a novel influenza A virus is introduced into the human population. 'Novel' in this context is to be understood as a virus that mankind has little or no pre-existing immunity against.

If a person or an animal is doubly infected by strains of different subtypes, this provides a chance for reassortment of the eight gene segments from each virus. In theory, this could generate 2^8, or 256, combinations. During the process of genetic reassortment, the HA gene, and also occasionally the NA gene, can be replaced, with or without the introduction of one or more of the other six gene segments from the other virus. If one of the parent viruses is of a subtype to which man has no prior immunity, we may face a situation where a 'new' virus with one or two novel surface antigens could be seeded into the human population. Experimentally, the reassortment mechanism has been used for a long time in the laboratory for generating 'seed' virus for vaccine production by doubly infecting embryonated eggs with a field strain and a well-characterized laboratory strain with good growth potential (typically the PR8 virus); from the resulting mixture of viruses it is possible to isolate a strain with surface antigens of the field strain and the other genes from the laboratory strain. Also, for live-attenuated influenza vaccines, strain reassortment is performed between a selected field isolate and a well-characterized attenuated laboratory strain, to generate an attenuated vaccine virus with surface proteins from the field isolate (see Chapter 9).

Whether reassortment is a frequent occurrence in the field is uncertain, but one assumes it to be a rare event. As an example, two human strains of the A/H3N2 and A/H1N1 subtypes must have recently reassorted (around 2001) to generate an

A/H1N2 subtype, which now is detected widely across the globe. Considering that the A/H3N2 and A/H1N1 subtypes have co-circulated in man since 1977, this chance reassortment appears to have taken approximately 25 years to have become apparent. However, it should be noted that other cases of human–human reassortment may have occurred previously but may have gone undetected and not be able to spread widely. In fact, the A/H1N2 subtype was detected sporadically in man in China in 1988 but did not seem to spread further.

Reverse genetics

In recent years a new biotechnology process called 'reverse genetics' has been developed, which can quickly and in a controlled fashion generate vaccine 'seed' viruses, for example from highly pathogenic avian viruses. Briefly, the two genes coding for the HA and NA surface antigens from the avian virus are added to the remaining six genes from a laboratory strain, such as the PR8 virus, to create a replication-competent virus in an approved cell line. Point mutations, for example in the HA gene, have been engineered at certain critical sites, creating a 'designer virus' suitable for vaccine use. This procedure can speed up the modification of a dangerous field virus into a licensed vaccine strain within a few weeks.

Consequences for the immune response

The various types of cross-immunity should be remembered as being extremely useful for the immune response, allowing earlier immunity to assist in neutralizing virus and clearing virus-infected cells (see 'Antigenic drift', above). If cross-reactions are within the same subtype, it is occasionally called 'homosubtypic immunity', recalling that the genetic and immunological ('antigenic') differences between the HAs from various subtypes (Tables 2.1 and 2.2) are quite substantial. We benefit frequently from cross-immunity between strains within a subtype. Previous winters' exposure to strains within the same subtype will to some extent modify and lessen the clinical impact once infected with the same or a closely related strain, thereby reducing the viral load in the airways and infectiousness to others in terms of virus quantity and duration of shedding. Thus, widespread cross-reactive herd immunity in the population will lessen the epidemiological impact in the community.

'Heterosubtypic immunity' is defined as immunity that transcends the subtype barrier. Such immunity could be mediated by unrecognized similar antigenic stretches in the HA molecules of the two subtypes, or, more likely, by immunity mediated by the more antigenically stable M1 and NP proteins, which are the main targets for the cytotoxic cellular immune response.

Measuring the antibody response

It was observed in the 1940s that influenza viruses had the capacity to bind to red blood cells (erythrocytes) and make them clump together. This phenomenon is used in a laboratory test called the haemagglutination-inhibition (HI) test. In simple terms, one takes serial dilutions of serum from a patient who has had an influenza infection or been vaccinated, and mixes these with a standardized quantity of virus, letting the virus and serum dilutions react for a certain time; into this mixture is then added a suspension of erythrocytes (e.g. from turkey or horse). If the serum sample contains antibodies able to bind to the virus particles, its ability to clump the red cells (haemagglutinate) could be blocked and can be measured as a titre, i.e. how many times a serum sample can be diluted before the virus can again haemagglutinate the red cells.

This test is still considered to be the 'gold standard' procedure for measuring the efficacy of influenza vaccines. A certain percentage of the vaccinees must have obtained a particular predefined level of HI antibodies in order for the vaccine to be licensed. A similar general procedure is used for virus-neutralization tests. Here one uses live virus, and the red cells are replaced by a laboratory cell line (frequently dog or monkey kidney cells). Again, non-neutralized virus will infect the cells and the presence of newly made virus can be measured.

The HI titre is used by the vaccine licensing authorities as a surrogate marker or correlate of immunity. The neutralizing antibodies are more relevant as they are measuring biological activity using live virus. However, the latter test is a complicated and time-consuming procedure, and is therefore mostly used in research settings. Also, the particular requirement for some avian HA subtypes that prefer the α-2,3 cellular receptor has been a particular challenge for both the HI test and the neutralization assays.

2.7 Pandemics

As we have seen, occasional transfer of avian influenza to man has happened many times, but in order to cause a pandemic there are more conditions to be met. According to a report by the WHO Secretariat for the 114th Session of the WHO Executive Board in April 2004, requirements for avian influenza to cause a pandemic are:

- A novel influenza virus (with a new HA subtype and possibly also a new NA) must emerge to which the general population has little or no immunity and against which no existing seasonal vaccine will be effective.
- The new virus must be able to replicate in man and cause disease.
- The new virus must be efficiently transmitted from one person to another; efficient human-to-human transmission is expressed as sustained chains of transmission causing community-wide outbreaks.

The initial report said 'against which no existing vaccine will be effective', however, much recent progress has been made in the preparation of A/H5N1 vaccines (see Chapter 9). Due to recent worldwide cases of a novel H1N1 virus, with a substantially antigenically different HA (swine), the pandemic definition requiring a 'new HA subtype' should be reconsidered.

The most devastating pandemic in recent history was the Spanish influenza of 1918. At that time the infectious agent was unknown. It took another 13 years before influenza virus was identified and could be grown experimentally in a laboratory, namely in 1931 (isolates from pigs) and 1933 (isolates from man). Several decades later and based on subsequent studies of sera from elderly people who had survived the pandemic, it was concluded that the virus must have belonged to the subtype

A/H1N1. The specific genetic make-up of the virus was unknown until very recently, when lung material from a 1918 victim found in a permafrost grave in Alaska, as well as from archived formalin-preserved sections of lung tissue from young soldiers who died of Spanish flu, was analysed. This was an impressive and highly significant scientific breakthrough.

In the following years, spurred by these findings and also by the A/H5N1 pandemic threat, the advances in influenza virology were many. A significant finding was that the 1918 virus most likely had an avian origin and that reassortment in a non-human host may not have been involved in the process. In other words, an avian virus had adapted directly to man without the need for reassortment in an intermediate host such as the pig. These features make the virological origins of the 1918 pandemic very different from those in 1957 and 1968, and may in turn explain the quantum difference in severity between 1918 on the one hand and 1957 and 1968 on the other. Finally, this finding defines the serious pandemic threat currently posed by A/H5N1 'bird flu' (see Chapters 3 and 4).

Based on the published genetic sequences of the 1918 flu, it was reconstructed by reverse genetics and tested in animal models. These studies confirmed what the doctors in the field had seen, namely that the virus was highly lethal, replicated rapidly in patients' lungs and frequently also spread to other organs. Figure 2.3 shows the various modes of generating pandemic strains. What specific properties of the virus made the 1918 virus so lethal to people? We still do not know. The scientific consensus is, however, that influenza virus pathogenicity is a multigenetic phenomenon involving many of the ten virus-coded proteins. Of particular relevance are the properties of the HA molecule. Highly pathogenic avian influenza (HPAI), i.e. the subtypes A/H5 and A/H7 ('fowl plague'), all have a polybasic cleavage point in the HA, the so-called 'promiscuous site'. In man, on the other hand, influenza pathogenicity may not directly be dependent upon this special feature. Recent zoonotic cases of infections with the avian A/H5N1, frequently associated with an extremely high mortality, have raised global awareness that a pandemic could be imminent. But antigenic novelty per se is not enough; the virus must also undergo other changes so it can spread easily from one person to the next. Only very few cases of human-to-human spread of A/H5N1 have so far been documented, and these are generally confined to instances of close family-like contacts. Some will say this is sheer luck, whereas others will say it shows that the A/H5N1 virus, having sporadically infected people since 1997, will never acquire such a capacity. We do not know, of course, and it is therefore prudent to prepare for such a situation.

2.8 Summary Points

- Antibodies against HA will bind to the virus and prevent it binding to the host cell, i.e. the antibodies are neutralizing. Antibodies to NA will typically block or reduce the release of newly made virus particles from an already infected cell, i.e. these antibodies will dampen the replication of virus and thus reduce the clinical symptoms and how contagious an infected individual is to others.
- The drugs amantadine and rimantadine interfere with the function of the M2 protein (the ion channel) located in the viral membrane (hence are known as M2-channel blockers). As a consequence, genetic material from the virus cannot

enter the cell and take advantage of the cellular machinery, and the replication cycle comes to a halt. The neuraminidase-inhibitor drugs block the function of the viral NA enzyme and thus inhibit the release of newly made virus particles from an already infected cell.

- Cell-mediated immunity will not block the initial infection but rather destroy virus-infected cells. There is a reciprocal cooperation between the humoral (antibody-generating) and cellular (cytotoxic T-cells) arms of the immune response, thus strengthening and modifying both.

- Immunological memory is the adaptive immunity's ability to respond quicker and stronger to a subsequent stimulation by foreign material. This foreign material can be a new infection with an identical or related virus. When we are 'primed', i.e. have experienced an earlier encounter with an infectious agent or a vaccine, the memory so generated will help us combat a subsequent infection much more efficiently.

- A pre-pandemic vaccine is given in anticipation of an imminent pandemic. It is presumed, and hoped, that the pandemic virus will be closely related to the vaccine virus, so that the vaccine-immunological memory thus generated by the pre-pandemic vaccine will lessen the clinical impact when the pandemic virus strikes, thus giving fewer cases of severe illness, hospitalizations and deaths.

Further Reading

Association of Microbiologists (1998) *The facts about... influenza.* http://www.amm.co.uk/newamm/files/factsabout/fa_flu.htm (accessed May 2009).

Center for Infectious Disease Research & Policy (2009) *Pandemic Influenza. Latest News.* http://www.cidrap.umn.edu/cidrap/content/influenza/panflu/index.html (accessed May 2009).

Centers for Disease Control and Prevention (2009) *Seasonal Influenza. Vaccinate Your Children.* http://www.cdc.gov/flu/protect/children.htm (accessed May 2009).

European Influenza Surveillance Network (2009) http://www.ecdc.europa.eu/en/activities/surveillance/EISN/Pages/home.aspx (accessed May 2009).

European Scientific Working Group on Influenza (2009) *ESWI Flucentre.* Influenza knowledge centre for healthcare workers, homepage. http://www.flucentre.org/ (accessed May 2009).

Frank, S.A. (2002) Experimental evolution: influenza. In: *Immunology and Evolution of Infectious Diseases*, Chapter 13. http://www.ncbi.nlm.nih.gov/bookshelf/br.fcgi?book=infdis&part=A213#A214 (accessed May 2009).

Microbiology and Immunology On-line (continuously updated) University of South Carolina, School of Medicine. http://pathmicro.med.sc.edu/book/immunol-sta.htm (accessed May 2009).

Taubenberger, J.K., Hultin, J.V. and Morens, D.M. (2007) *Discovery and characterization of the 1918 pandemic influenza virus in historical context.* PubMedCentral 2008, 22 May. National Institutes of Health Public Access (USA). *Antiviral Therapy* 12, 581–591.

US Department of Health and Human Services and National Institutes of Health (2003) *Understanding the Immune System. How It Works.* NIH Publication No. 03-5423. http://www.niaid.nih.gov/publications/immune/the_immune_system.pdf (accessed May 2009).

World Health Organization (2009) *Epidemic and Pandemic Alert and Response (EPR). Avian influenza.* http://www.who.int/csr/disease/avian_influenza/en/index.html (accessed May 2009).

3 Avian and Animal Influenza: Manifestations in Man

C. SELLWOOD

- Which subtypes of influenza can be found in birds?
- What other animal reservoirs are there for influenza viruses?
- What is the difference between low-pathogenic and high-pathogenic avian influenza?
- Why is A/H5N1 of such concern?
- What are the particular concerns in an area where A/H5N1 is endemic in birds?

3.1 Introduction

Avian influenza is a disease of birds caused by the influenza A virus. The natural reservoir for such viruses is wild waterfowl, predominantly ducks and geese, although the viruses have been isolated from birds of over 18 families. The viruses can circulate undetected in waterfowl populations as infected birds usually remain healthy. Individual birds remain infected for about 1 month, during which time the virus replicates in the gastrointestinal tract and is excreted in extremely high levels in faeces. Large congregations of wild birds prior to migration provide perfect conditions for transmission and mixing of avian influenza viruses and ensure the animal reservoir is maintained.

Avian influenza has been recognized in poultry for over a century, although the disease was associated with the influenza A virus only in the 1950s. Domestic poultry flocks are especially vulnerable to infections, with significant repercussions for human livelihoods and the potential for human health implications. However, transmission to people in close contact with poultry or other birds occurs rarely and has been reported only with certain subtypes of avian influenza, particularly A/H5, A/H7 and, to a lesser extent, A/H9 viruses. This chapter discusses avian influenza in birds and man, as well as influenza A in other mammalian species.

3.2 Avian Influenza in Wild and Domesticated Birds

Avian influenza is regularly detected in wild birds through routine surveillance, and all of the 16 haemagglutinin (HA) and nine neuraminidase (NA) subtypes of influenza viruses are known to infect species of wild waterfowl. Most avian influenza viruses cause little or no disease and circulate undetected; they are classified as low-pathogenic avian influenza (LPAI) owing to the low fatality rate inflicted on infected domestic poultry.

©CAB International 2010. *Introduction to Pandemic Influenza*
(eds J.S. Nguyen-Van-Tam and C. Sellwood)

LPAI is a common disease in domestic poultry, where the only signs of illness may be decreased egg production, reduced appetite, ruffled feathers, swollen heads or mild respiratory symptoms. Outbreaks can be so mild they go undetected or are not thought to be due to influenza. Only A/H9N2 can be described as endemic in poultry populations, particularly in certain parts of the Middle East.

If either an A/H5 or an A/H7 LPAI virus infects poultry it can remain in a low-pathogenic form or it may mutate and be associated with rapidly spreading large outbreaks of high mortality. In these instances the virus is described as 'highly pathogenic avian influenza' (HPAI). Only A/H5 and A/H7 subtypes are recognized to occur as HPAI. This form of the virus was first recognized in Italy in 1878, and is extremely contagious in domestic poultry and rapidly fatal. The first recorded instance of an LPAI virus mutating into a highly pathogenic form occurred in Scotland, UK in 1959. HPAI viruses have a characteristic set of basic amino acids in the haemagglutinin cleavage site which differentiates them from all other avian influenza viruses and is associated with their high virulence and mortality rate. However, there is no automatic correlation between the high or low pathogenic status of A/H5 and A/H7 viruses and the pattern of disease they cause in man; HPAI sometimes causes mild conjunctivitis in a human host (e.g. A/H7N7) whereas LPAI has been associated with respiratory illness sufficient to cause hospitalization (e.g. A/H7N2).

HPAI in poultry is characterized by the sudden onset of severe disease, rapid spread, and a mortality rate that can approach 100% within 48 h. Birds often die on the day that symptoms appear. HPAI causes respiratory symptoms (like LPAI) but these are accompanied by massive internal haemorrhaging as the virus invades multiple organs and tissues, and cyanosis, diarrhoea and death. In some outbreaks, other avian viruses such as Norfolk Disease have been considered as possible causes, however, the rapid spread and high fatality rate tend to be highly indicative of HPAI, which is then confirmed through laboratory testing.

Prior to the emergence of A/H5N1 in 1997, outbreaks of HPAI in poultry were relatively uncommon (Table 3.1). Recent HPAI outbreaks have occurred across the

Table 3.1. Significant poultry outbreaks of avian influenza.

Year	Country	Strain	Comments
1983–1984	Pennsylvania, USA	A/H5N2	17 million birds culled at a cost of US$65 million
1992–1995	Mexico	A/H5N2	Four years to bring under control
1997	Hong Kong	A/H5N1	All poultry culled to bring outbreak under control, 18 human cases, including six fatalities
2003	Netherlands	A/H7N3	Widespread poultry culling and separation from wild birds, over 80 human cases, including one fatality
2004	Canada	A/H7N3	17 million poultry culled, two mild human cases
2003 onwards	Global	A/H5N1	Widespread poultry outbreaks across South-east Asia, Middle East, Africa and Southern Europe. Over 400 human cases, 60% fatality rate

globe, in countries such as Canada, Hong Kong SAR, Italy, Mexico, the Netherlands, Pakistan, South Africa, the UK and the USA. The outbreaks have ranged in size from a single flock to a global scale as seen with HPAI A/H5N1, which is now considered endemic in poultry and wild birds in many parts of Asia, Africa and the Middle East. HPAI is now endemic in commercial and backyard poultry in Indonesia and Egypt, and the number of smaller outbreaks restricted to one premise or farm is difficult to quantify but likely to be extremely large.

It was previously thought that wild birds were infected only by LPAI strains while HPAI was a disease of poultry, however, HPAI A/H5N1 has proved to be capable of infecting and killing wild birds. It is of particular concern that HPAI A/H5N1 has now been detected in migratory wild birds, thus indicating a means by which the virus can spread globally. In 2005, over 6000 migratory wild birds infected with the HPAI A/H5N1 virus died at the Qinghai Lake nature reserve in central China. Viruses that were virtually identical to the Qinghai Lake viruses were isolated in early 2006 from two fatal human cases of A/H5N1 in Turkey.

Figure 3.1 illustrates the major wild bird flyways which may provide a route for the dispersal of avian influenza viruses. Contact points between the flyways may aid dispersal between populations of migratory and non-migratory wild birds and between species within the different flyways. Within Europe, and for certain

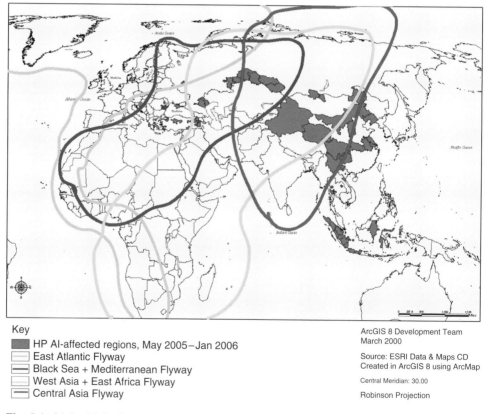

Key

HP AI-affected regions, May 2005–Jan 2006
East Atlantic Flyway
Black Sea + Mediterranean Flyway
West Asia + East Africa Flyway
Central Asia Flyway

ArcGIS 8 Development Team
March 2000

Source: ESRI Data & Maps CD
Created in ArcGIS 8 using ArcMap

Central Meridian: 30.00

Robinson Projection

Fig. 3.1. Major bird migration flyways. (Courtesy of the Global Animal Health Team, UK Department for the Environment, Food and Rural Affairs.)

C. Sellwood

species (e.g. ducks), flyways tend to be poorly defined. Migration occurs on a broad front, typically between a number of wetland staging areas. In the UK, more detailed analysis of bird migratory flyways, which are species-dependent, is carried out using the Migration Mapping Tool developed by the British Trust for Ornithology with funding from the UK Department for the Environment, Food and Rural Affairs (Defra), which allows risk analyses of how avian influenza might be dispersed along different routes within the context of known migration patterns for certain species.

Outbreaks of avian influenza, especially HPAI, can be devastating for the poultry industry and for farmers. An outbreak of HPAI A/H5N2 in the US state of Pennsylvania resulted in the destruction of more than 17 million birds at a cost of nearly US$65 million. The economic consequences of HPAI can be particularly significant in developing countries where poultry are an important source of income and food.

In assessing the risk to human health associated with an outbreak in birds, it is important to know which avian influenza virus is responsible. Based on currently available data, outbreaks caused by HPAI A/H5N1 and A/H7N7 are presently of the greatest concern for human health as these have both been associated with human deaths.

3.3   Influenza in Other Species

While avian influenza is widely recognized and reported in birds and man, influenza is known to be able to cause significant outbreaks of disease in other mammals including pigs, dogs, large and small cats, horses, seals, whales, mink and stone martens.

Pigs

Swine influenza is a highly contagious disease in pigs that is present in pig populations in all countries where these animals are reared. The disease can present with a variety of respiratory symptoms (such as coughing, sneezing and breathlessness), lethargy and reduced appetite. Although morbidity rates can reach 100%, recovery can be rapid and mortality is often low. As with human influenza, the infection can be complicated by secondary bacterial infections. The disease can cause a significant financial impact if the affected population is reared for commercial purposes, primarily because of an increase in the time needed to reach target weight.

Both epidemic and endemic swine influenza is known to occur in pig populations. In the epidemic form, the virus moves quickly throughout the population and resolves quickly, provided there are no complications such as secondary bacterial infections. In the endemic form, the clinical signs of swine influenza can be less obvious, while some animals may not even show the traditional symptoms.

The subtypes of influenza most commonly identified in pigs are the same as those that were responsible for the three influenza pandemics of the 20th century (namely, A/H1N1, A/H2N2 and A/H3N2) although other subtypes have been identified in pigs, including A/H1N7, A/H3N1, A/H4N6 and A/H9N2.

Pigs have often been described as 'mixing vessels' for influenza A viruses owing to their capacity to be co-infected by human and avian influenza viruses. This is due to the presence of receptors in their respiratory tract to which avian, human and swine influenza viruses can bind, thus enabling the viruses to recombine and give rise to novel strains. It is believed that this mixing vessel characteristic of pigs was responsible for the evolution of the pandemic influenza A/H2N2 and A/H3N2 viruses in 1957 and 1968, whereby avian viruses acquired new genetic material.

Human infections with swine influenza can occur and a limited number of deaths have been reported. For example, an outbreak of swine influenza A/H1N1 in the USA in 1977 affected over 200 people and caused one fatality (Chapter 4).

Dogs – USA and Thailand

Influenza A/H3N8 is a recognized respiratory pathogen in dogs, and has been associated with outbreaks of acute respiratory disease since it was first identified in US greyhounds in 2004. It has subsequently been identified in greyhounds in other countries and in other dog breeds in the USA.

A fatal infection of avian influenza A/H5N1 has also been reported in a domestic dog, where a 12-month-old dog died following consumption of an A/H5N1-infected duck carcass during an outbreak in Thailand. The dog developed a high fever, increased breathing rate (panting) and lethargy 5 days after eating the duck carcass, and died the following day. A/H5N1 virus was subsequently isolated from the lung, liver and kidney of the dog, as well as in the urine, indicating widespread infection.

Cats – tigers, leopards and domestic cats

Influenza is not generally thought of as pathogenic in domestic cats. However, domestic cats were experimentally infected with A/H3N2 from man, A/H7N3 from turkeys and A/H7N7 from seals in the 1970s and 1980s. Although the cats did not display physical signs of disease, temporary virus excretion and fever were reported. There have been anecdotal reports of fatal HPAI A/H5N1 infections in domestic cats in Asia in 2003–2004, which were subsequently experimentally confirmed. Domestic cats were symptomatically infected through intra-tracheal inoculation and by feeding on dead chicks infected with HPAI A/H5N1. The infected cats then excreted virus and transmitted the infection to sentinel cats placed in the same cages.

Influenza had not been widely reported to affect wild cats. However in January 2004, HPAI A/H5N1 caused severe pneumonia, fever and respiratory distress in two captive tigers and leopards fed infected chicken carcasses in a zoo in Thailand. All four cats subsequently died.

In October 2004, animals in a different tiger zoo in Thailand were affected by HPAI A/H5N1. The population of 441 tigers was housed in three separate zones (breeder, nursery and grower) and the outbreak initially involved 16 tigers aged 6 to 24 months in the grower zone. Within 3 days, five animals had died and 14 others showed clinical symptoms, including high fever and respiratory distress. Although the infection did not spread to the breeder or nursery zones, the outbreak continued to spread among tigers in the grower zone until eventually nearly 150 cats were eutha-nized or died due to A/H5N1 infection. While the initial infection is believed to have been introduced through feeding of infected poultry carcases, there was also evidence of horizontal tiger-to-tiger transmission.

The detection of A/H5N1 in wild cats increases the range of hosts for the influenza virus and may have potential future implications for the spread of disease to human populations who live with domestic cats.

Horses – Australia, 2007

Equine influenza is an acute, contagious respiratory disease of domestic horses, donkeys and mules caused by A/H7N7 and A/H3N8 viruses. Clinical signs include fever and a harsh, dry cough that spread rapidly among susceptible animals; however, partially immune vaccinated animals may be infected without showing these symptoms. Man has only rarely been infected with equine influenza, and the cases where this has occurred have been subclinical.

Equine influenza is of low concern to most countries, and is endemic in many including the UK and the USA; however, a widespread outbreak of A/H3N8 in Australia that started in 2007 had a significant impact in that country. The outbreak started in August 2007, following the movement of 13 infected horses from Japan to Melbourne, Australia, and rapidly spread throughout New South Wales and Queensland. Breaches of the quarantine protocols in both Japan and Australia caused the outbreak and subsequent spread of disease.

Following the identification of equine influenza, the Australian authorities implemented a rigorous programme of control and eradication including stopping horse movement across the country, strict bio-security measures, and vaccination in infected areas and surrounding buffer zones; all supported by extensive surveillance across the country. The outbreak was successfully restricted to parts of the southeastern states of New South Wales and Queensland – while all other Australian states and territories remained free from disease. Nevertheless, the outbreak almost destroyed the multi-million-dollar horse breeding industry in Australia. The final cases in the outbreak were reported in December 2007, and Australia was finally declared free from equine influenza 6 months later in June 2008. The Australian government estimated that the outbreak cost the racing and breeding industries more than AU$1 billion.

3.4   Avian Influenza in Man

A range of avian influenza subtypes have caused illness in man (Table 3.2). LPAI A/H9N2 in Hong Kong caused mild illness in two children in 1999 and in one child in December 2003. A 2-month-old girl was infected with A/H9N2 in China in December 2008.

A widespread outbreak of HPAI A/H7N7 in poultry in the Netherlands that began in February 2003 led to over 450 reports of illness (mainly conjunctivitis and minor respiratory symptoms) in poultry workers, farmers and their immediate families, along with evidence of limited person-to-person transmission. Of the 450 people

Table 3.2. Some recent documented human infections with avian influenza viruses.

Year	Country	Subtype	Pathogenicity	Cases
1995	UK	A/H7N7	–	One mild case of conjunctivitis
1997	Hong Kong	A/H5N1	HPAI	Eighteen cases (six fatal)
1999	Hong Kong	A/H9N2	LPAI	Two mild cases, children
2003	Hong Kong	A/H9N2	LPAI	One mild case, child
2003	Netherlands	A/H7N7	HPAI	Eighty-nine cases; mainly conjunctivitis or mild respiratory symptoms (one fatality)
2004	Canada	A/H7N3	LPAI	Two mild cases
2006	UK	A/H7N3	LPAI	One mild case conjunctivitis
2007	China	A/H9N2	LPAI	One mild case, child
2007	UK	A/H7N2	LPAI	Four cases (three hospitalized with respiratory symptoms)
2008	China	A/H9N2	LPAI	One mild case
Late 2003 to present	South-east Asia, Middle East, Africa, Europe	A/H5N1	HPAI	Over 400 cases (over 60% fatal) severe respiratory symptoms and multi-organ failure in most fatal cases, diarrhoea common in children

reporting illness, there were 89 confirmed cases of A/H7N7 infection, including one death from an acute respiratory illness 2 months later. The outbreak was bought under control by thorough and widespread culling of poultry in the Netherlands, as well as measures to isolate poultry from wild birds.

An outbreak of HPAI A/H7N3 occurred in poultry in British Columbia, Canada in 2004 that necessitated the culling of 17 million birds. There were two human cases of illness (LPAI A/H7N3 was detected in one of the cases, HPAI A/H7N3 in the other) both of which presented with mild symptoms (conjunctivitis in one and mild respiratory symptoms in the other). A separate outbreak of LPAI A/H7N3 in poultry in the east of England in May 2006 caused one human case of conjunctivitis.

In May 2007, LPAI A/H7N2 was identified in Wales and north-west England, in birds purchased at a livestock market. Four cases of human disease were associated with this outbreak, three of which were hospitalized on clinical grounds with influenza-like symptoms. Previously only two unrelated human cases of conjunctivitis had been reported in the literature as due to this virus.

However, the few cases of human illness described above associated with A/H7 and A/H9 strains, mainly mild respiratory symptoms or conjunctivitis, are greatly over-shadowed by the extent of avian and human disease caused by HPAI A/H5N1 since it first came to notice in 1997.

The A/H5N1 crisis and its special significance

Since 1997, and with increasing focus from 2003, HPAI A/H5N1 has come to public attention as having infected and killed large numbers of poultry and wild water birds

C. Sellwood

across South-east Asia, parts of Africa and Eastern Europe. There have also been a number of associated human infections. At the time of writing, HPAI A/H5N1 has been responsible for over 400 human infections, of which about 60% have proved fatal. While it is by no means certain that this virus will cause the next human influenza pandemic, experts predict that the most likely source of the next pandemic will be South-east Asia and that A/H5N1 is currently a serious and credible contender. This is supported by evidence that the virus is undergoing a process of rapid genetic diversification and change, with ten phylogenetically distinct clades having already been described, of which three have been associated with disease in man.

Influenza A/H5N1 first came to worldwide attention in 1997 following a widespread outbreak in poultry in Hong Kong. Despite probable wide-scale exposure of the local human population to the infected poultry, clinical illness was extremely rare. Only eighteen human cases were associated with the outbreak, however, all were severe enough to be hospitalized and six of the cases subsequently died. There was no evidence of transmission between people, and all 18 cases had contact with live or recently killed birds. The Hong Kong authorities undertook drastic control measures; Hong Kong's entire poultry population, estimated at around 1.5 million birds, was culled within 3 days in order to stamp out the virus, and rules were introduced around selling and handling live birds. Human infections stopped, suggesting that these measures had been successful, until the virus re-emerged elsewhere in South-east Asia in late 2003.

The first human cases associated with the current outbreaks were reported in Vietnam in December 2003. Subsequently, a pre-dated case was reported in China, in a member of the military based in Beijing in November 2003. Human cases of A/H5N1 have since been reported from countries across the world with the majority of cases in Indonesia and Thailand. As of the start of 2009, sixteen countries had reported human case of avian influenza A/H5N1 – Azerbaijan, Bangladesh, Cambodia, China, Djibouti, Egypt, Indonesia, Iraq, Lao People's Democratic Republic, Myanmar, Nepal, Nigeria, Pakistan, Thailand, Turkey and Vietnam. Surveillance and control of avian influenza can be particularly hard in these countries due to the size and distribution of the poultry population. For example, there are approximately 4.6 billion chickens, 700 million ducks and 300 million geese spread across China in varying ratios. The majority of duck populations are found in southern and south-eastern China, and geese are found in the drier north-eastern and extreme western part of China, while chickens are everywhere that people live, particularly in urban areas, where backyard farming is commonplace.

Almost all human cases of A/H5N1 have been attributed to direct exposure to infected birds, although limited, unsustained person-to-person spread cannot be excluded in a few cases in Indonesia and Thailand, where either co-exposure could not be ruled out or very close 'healthcare-like' care was given to an infected individual by other family members. Furthermore, although extensive studies have not yet been undertaken, the available data suggest that A/H5N1 is not causing undetected asymptomatic or mild cases on a wide scale. This is illustrated by the lack of evidence of seroconversion not only in the wider population, but also in healthcare workers caring for A/H5N1 patients and in cohorts of poultry workers. One paper which identified a supposedly high frequency of mild A/H5N1 infections in Vietnam was based on a retrospective questionnaire and seriously flawed in its conclusions because the findings were unsupported by serological evidence of infection.

A/H5N1 in man

Most human cases of A/H5N1 have been in people who were previously healthy, with 90% of patients aged 40 years or younger, with the average age being around 18 years; there have been noticeably fewer cases in older adults. This age-specific correlation may reflect exposure opportunity (frequency of exposure) related to the fact that husbandry of backyard flocks is frequently devolved to younger members of the extended family. In line with this, the death rate is highest in patients aged 10–19 years and lowest in cases aged 50 years or over. This could reflect a cytokine-mediated response to A/H5N1 infection in younger subjects (the so-called 'cytokine storm'); or different infectious doses received by age; or possibly a degree of background immunity to A/H5N1 infection in older subjects (see early A/H5N1 vaccine trials in Chapter 9). Handling sick or dead poultry in the week prior to onset of illness is typically associated with infection. To date (2009) there have been no cases associated with travellers or tourists visiting affected areas.

The majority of cases have been in isolated individuals, however, clusters of at least two epidemiologically linked cases have been identified, and collectively account for approximately 25% of all cases. The majority of clusters have consisted of two or three blood-related family members, indicating the potential for some underlying genetic susceptibility, although this has not been confirmed. The occurrence of clusters of cases is usually associated with common exposure to infected poultry, although in some cases it has not been possible to rule out the possibility of limited person-to-person transmission through close healthcare worker-like contact. The largest cluster was reported in Indonesia in 2006, where the initial case infected six blood relatives and subsequently one other family member.

Human cases of A/H5N1 have typically been significantly more severe than seasonal influenza. Cases have been characterized by severe illness, including fever, shortness of breath, cough, and severe pneumonia (in about 80% of cases), which often progresses rapidly to acute respiratory distress syndrome. Diarrhoea has been reported more frequently than with seasonal influenza, especially among children, and has often been reported before respiratory symptoms have started. Organ failure is also comparatively common, particularly liver dysfunction. The time of onset of illness to death is typically 9–10 days.

As awareness of the disease, early medical attention and antiviral treatment have increased, the clinical course of illness in patients has altered; for example, there have been fewer reports of gastrointestinal symptoms since 2005. Influenza A/H5N1 has varying susceptibility to the M2-inhibitor drugs (rimantidine and amantadine) and to the neuraminidase-inhibitor drug (oseltamivir) depending on the virus clade. Some strains are fully resistant to the M2 inhibitors, while variants resistant to oseltamivir have emerged during treatment; the latter is associated with fatal outcome. Nevertheless, early treatment with oseltamivir is recommended, and there is evidence that early treatment improves survival rates. Oseltamivir-resistant strains of A/H5N1 tend to be sensitive to the other licensed neuraminidase inhibitor, zanamivir, although to date it has not been widely used, in part because it is an inhaled drug and its effectiveness in clinical practice (as opposed to *in vitro* activity) against A/H5N1 is not clearly known. The role of antiviral drugs and antibiotics is discussed more extensively in Chapter 8.

C. Sellwood

3.5 Managing the Human and Public Health Consequences of Avian Influenza in Poultry

As described earlier, LPAI viruses regularly circulate undetected in wild bird populations, however, HPAI has also been detected in these species. While little can or needs to be done about LPAI in wild birds, measures should be taken when HPAI is detected in order to reduce the contact between wild and domestic birds. These interventions can include measures to isolate populations through housing domestic birds and preventing wild birds accessing domestic birds' water or feed supplies (e.g. through the use of nets and indoor housing). For example, during an outbreak of avian influenza or in periods of increased risk in the UK, it is recommended that all free-range and backyard poultry is housed.

Outbreaks of avian influenza in poultry should be dealt with promptly, especially A/H5 and A/H7 subtypes, as LPAI viruses from these can mutate into HPAI. Poultry outbreaks of HPAI can be addressed through rapid culling and disposal of carcasses, implementing strict bio-security measures such as quarantining and disinfecting premises and equipment, and restricting live poultry movement. This is reasonably easy to implement on large commercial farms, where birds are generally housed and there are existing bio-security processes. It is not so easy where birds are free-range or exist as small rural backyard flocks; this may have contributed to the endemicity of A/H5N1 in South-east Asia.

Where culling is impractical or ineffective, vaccination can be used as an additional emergency measure, however, this should not be implemented without thorough consideration. Although it can be successful in large-scale commercial settings, it is too expensive to be applied routinely to backyard flocks in resource-poor settings. Furthermore, while vaccines may be used in conjunction with other control measures to damp down infection in an endemic area, they may have limited use in sporadic outbreaks as their use can increase longevity of viraemia in infected birds and induce short-lived immunity. Finally, the vaccine requires regular updating to ensure that it is closely matched to circulating strains, adding to the cost of such programmes, and use of vaccines that do not match the outbreak strain may make the situation worse. Vaccinated birds can be infected and continue to shed virus while remaining well and appearing disease-free, thus necessitating the use of unvaccinated sentinel birds.

As well as being harder to control than commercial outbreaks of avian influenza, outbreaks in backyard flocks are associated with an increased risk of human exposure and infection. These flocks can come into regular close contact with wild birds and so be easily exposed to a range of avian influenza viruses. Backyard flocks are often highly valuable to their owners and frequently enter homes while scavenging or are brought in at night for protection, thus providing increased opportunities for transmission of the virus to the human population. Additionally, children may treat birds as pets and play with them, while cock-fighting is another pastime where transmission to people can occur.

Deaths in backyard flocks are common, and where poultry is the main source of food or income and resources and education are limited, birds which have died or appear to be ill may be eaten rather than disposed of. While cooking is known to inactivate the virus, there have been human cases where infection has been associated with slaughtering, de-feathering, evisceration and preparing birds for consumption, all of which provide increased opportunities and easy routes for the virus to spread from infected poultry to man.

Although the majority of cases can be linked with direct or environmental contact with infected birds, there are some instances where the route of infection is less clear-cut. In such cases, transmission may have occurred through exposure to faecal dust/contaminated blood when walking through live poultry markets, consuming raw poultry products (although there is a roughly tenfold higher concentration of the virus in the organs of infected poultry compared with skeletal muscle, virus transmission is still possible through this route), contact with faeces in fertilizer or when cleaning poultry living areas, or even in rare and unproven circumstances, swimming/bathing in heavily virus-contaminated waterways.

3.6   Pandemic Preparedness

Avian influenza A/H5N1 is a clear and present danger to human health in terms of its current lethality to the human population and its potential to cause a future pandemic, however, it would be short-sighted to become over-focused on this one virus to the exclusion of other avian influenza viruses and previous human pandemic subtypes such as A/H2N2. Pandemic planning needs to be flexible and applicable to any subtype or strain of influenza that may arise. With the exception of the development of subtype-specific A/H5N1 vaccines (Chapter 9) that may play a role should A/H5N1 achieve eventual pandemic status, all other interventions being developed and considered are applicable to any subtype of influenza.

Focus Box 3.1. The main differences between avian, seasonal and pandemic influenza.

Avian influenza is a common disease of birds caused by the influenza A virus, and is of concern to human health when it jumps the species barrier to infect the human population. This is an event that occurs relatively infrequently when placed in the context of the number of contacts people have with poultry and other bird species. Of these contacts, many either do not result in disease or cause mild influenza-like illness or non-respiratory symptoms such as conjunctivitis. Some avian influenza subtypes are able to cause significant illness in man, however, none of these has so far developed the ability to spread easily among the human population.

Seasonal influenza describes human disease due to influenza A subtypes that are already circulating in the human population or influenza B. Activity occurs year-round but has a clear seasonal pattern in the southern and northern hemispheres. Morbidity and mortality are highest in recognized at-risk groups such as the elderly, the very young or those with underlying risk conditions.

Pandemic influenza occurs when a novel influenza virus spreads in the human population, causing widespread and significant illness on a global scale. Pandemic influenza can start at any time of year, attack any age group, and causes far greater mortality and morbidity than seasonal influenza.

C. Sellwood

3.7　Summary Points

- Subtypes containing all 16 known haemagglutinin and nine neuraminidase antigens are known to occur in wild birds. A/H5N1, various A/H7 subtypes and A/H9N2 are of particular concern for human health and economic prosperity.
- Influenza viruses have been detected in a range of bird species, from wild aquatic shore birds to domestic poultry, as well as in a variety of mammalian species such as pigs, horses, dogs, large and domestic cats, stone martens and seals.
- The difference between LPAI and HPAI refers to the different pathogenicity of the virus in poultry, not in man. LPAI is a common disease in poultry that is often so mild as to go undetected. Key signs of illness include reduced egg production, reduced appetite or mild respiratory symptoms. HPAI in poultry is a severe disease with sudden onset, rapid spread and a very high mortality rate. HPAI causes respiratory symptoms in poultry that are accompanied by internal haemorrhaging, cyanosis, diarrhoea and death.
- Avian influenza A/H5N1 is of concern to human health because it is widespread in birds and poultry and lethal in man. Should this particular virus develop the ability to spread efficiently between people there is a significant risk of a severe pandemic occurring.
- In areas where A/H5N1 is endemic in wild birds and/or domestic poultry, there is an increased risk of the virus being transmitted to the human population, with the associated risk of the virus mutating to be able to spread from person to person.

Further Reading

Abdel-Ghafar, A.N., Chotpitayasunondh, T., Gao, Z., Hayden, F.G., Nguyen, D.H., de Jong, M.D., Naghdaliyev, A., Peiris, J.S., Shindo, N., Soeroso, S. and Uyeki, T.M.; Writing Committee of the Second World Health Organization Consultation on Clinical Aspects of Human Infection with Avian Influenza A (H5N1) Virus (2008) Update on avian influenza A (H5N1) infection in humans. *New England Journal of Medicine* 358, 261–273.

Beigel, J.H., Farrar, J., Han, A.M., Hayden, F.G., Hyer, R., de Jong, M.D., Lochindarat, S., Nguyen, T.K., Nguyen, T.H., Tran, T.H., Touch, S. and Yuen, K.Y.; Writing Committee of the World Health Organization (WHO) Consultation on Human Influenza A/H5 (2005) Avian influenza A (H5N1) infection in humans. *New England Journal of Medicine* 353, 1374–1385. Erratum in *New England Journal of Medicine* (2006) 354, 884.

Chan, M.C., Cheung, C.Y., Chui, W.H., Tsao, S.W., Nicholls, J.M., Chan, Y.O., Chan, R.W., Long, H.T., Poon, L.L., Guan, Y. and Peiris, J.S. (2005) Proinflammatory cytokine responses induced by influenza A (H5N1) viruses in primary human alveolar and bronchial epithelial cells. *Respiratory Research* 6, 135.

Crick, H.Q.P., Atkinson, P.W., Newson, S.E., Robinson, R.A., Snow, L., Balmer, D.E., Chamberlain, D.E., Clark, J.A., Clark, N.A., Cranswick, P.A., Cromie, R.L., Hughes, B., Grantham, M.J., Lee, R. and Musgrove, A.J. (2006) *Avian Influenza Incursion Analysis (through wild birds).* BTO Research Report No. 448. http://www.bto.org/research/reports/Avian_flu.pdf (accessed May 2009).

Koopmans, M., Wilbrink, B., Conyn, M., Natrop, G., van der Nat, H., Vennema, H., Meijer, A., van Steenbergen, J., Fouchier, R., Osterhaus, A. and Bosman, A. (2004) Transmission of H7N7 avian influenza virus to human beings during a large outbreak in commercial poultry farms in the Netherlands. *Lancet* 363, 587–593.

Sabirovic, M., Hall, S., Wilesmith, J. and Coulson, N. (2007) *Highly Pathogenic Avian Influenza – H5N1: Recent Developments in the EU and the Likelihood of the Introduction into Great Britain by Wild Birds, Version 1*. Department for the Environment, Food and Rural Affairs, London.

Smith, G.J., Naipospos, T.S., Nguyen, T.D., de Jong, M.D., Vijaykrishna, D., Usman, T.B., Hassan, S.S., Nguyen, T.V., Dao, T.V., Bui, N.A., Leung, Y.H., Cheung, C.L., Rayner, J.M., Zhang, J.X., Zhang, L.J., Poon, L.L., Li, K.S., Nguyen, V.C., Hien, T.T., Farrar, J., Webster, R.G., Chen, H., Peiris, J.S. and Guan, Y. (2006) Evolution and adaptation of H5N1 influenza virus in avian and human hosts in Indonesia and Vietnam. *Virology* 350, 258–268.

Webster, R.G. and Hay, A.J. (1998) The H5N1 influenza outbreak in Hong Kong: a test of pandemic preparedness. In: Nicholson, K.G., Webster, R.G. and Hay, A.J. (eds) *Textbook of Influenza*. Blackwell Science Ltd, Oxford, pp. 561–565.

World Health Organization (2005) *Epidemic and Pandemic Alert and Response (EPR). Avian influenza: assessing the pandemic threat*. http://www.who.int/csr/disease/influenza/WHO_CDS_2005_29/en/index.html (accessed May 2009).

World Health Organization Global Influenza Program Surveillance Network (2005) Evolution of H5N1 avian influenza viruses in Asia. *Emerging Infectious Diseases* 11, 1515–1521.

4 Brief History and Epidemiological Features of Pandemic Influenza

C. SELLWOOD

- Which influenza A subtypes caused the pandemics of the 20th century?
- What was the worst pandemic?
- Have pandemics occurred in earlier history?
- What can we predict about the epidemiology of the next pandemic?
- What influenza viruses are of concern at the present time?

4.1 Introduction

An influenza pandemic is an outbreak of influenza encompassing the whole world. It is a rare but recurrent event that occurs when a new influenza virus emerges that is able to spread easily from person to person, and against which people have little or no immunity. The resulting global outbreak affects many more people than a regular seasonal influenza epidemic, and has the potential to cause far greater morbidity and mortality. This chapter discusses pandemics that have occurred previously and introduces the concept of pandemic preparedness upon which subsequent chapters focus.

4.2 Prerequisites for Pandemic Influenza

In order for a pandemic to occur, four key criteria must be met:

1. A new influenza A virus unrelated to the circulating pre-pandemic viruses must emerge or evolve and circulate in people.
2. There must be little or no pre-existing immunity in the global population to the new virus.
3. The new virus must cause significant clinical illness.
4. The virus must be able to spread efficiently from person to person.

4.3 Pandemics before the 20th Century

The three influenza pandemics of the 20th century (in 1918, 1957 and 1968, see later) are well reported and it is from studying these that much of our planning and preparedness for a future pandemic is based. Pandemics prior to 1918 are less well documented, but still help to inform thinking and are of interest.

Table 4.1. Influenza pandemics since 1580.

Year	Affected areas	Origin	Subtype
1580	Europe, North America, Africa	Asia	Unknown
1729–1733	Europe, Americas, Russia	Russia	Unknown
1781–1782	Europe, North America, Russia, China, India	Russia/China	Unknown
1830–1833	Europe, North America, Russia, China, India	China	Unknown
1889–1892	Global	Russia	A/H2
1898–1900	Europe, Americas, Australia	Unknown	A/H3
1918–1920	Global	USA/China	A/H1N1
1957–1958	Global	China	A/H2N2
1968–1969	Global	China	A/H3N2

Influenza pandemics have probably occurred periodically throughout history. The first may have been identified in 412 BC by Hippocrates, and accounts of 'epidemic fever' – rapidly spreading outbreaks of febrile respiratory illness that caused a high excess mortality – appear in historical texts dating back to the 1500s. Two large outbreaks of influenza in 1510 and 1557 may have been pandemics, although the first widely recognized pandemic occurred in 1580 (Table 4.1). In relation to all of these historical writings it should always be borne in mind that there is no supporting virological evidence whatsoever and only limited evidence for the period between 1889 and 1918.

From 1500 until the mid-19th century

1580

The first recognized pandemic started in Asia in the summer of 1580 and within 6 months had spread to Africa and Europe, and then on to North America. Illness rates were high, and a common feature of future influenza pandemics was reported in the UK: the occurrence of multiple waves of infection – in the summer and the autumn of that year.

1729–1733

The first recognized pandemic of the 1700s occurred from 1729 to 1733. This pandemic originated in the spring of 1729 in Russia; within 6 months all of Europe was affected and in 3 years the whole world. There were two waves of infection, the latter more severe than the first, and the second wave in Europe coincided with the first wave in North America. This pandemic could be described as two separate unrelated outbreaks of influenza, the first in 1729–1730 being less severe, with a true pandemic in 1732–1733. However, the more accepted view is that there was a single pandemic covering the period, with a milder wave during which extensive 'seeding' of the virus preceded the more severe later waves caused by those seeding events. Regardless of whether this should be defined as one or two events, high death rates from influenza were reported across the globe throughout the period.

C. Sellwood

1781–1782

The second 18th-century pandemic started in autumn 1781 in China, and spread to Russia. The outbreak then spread west to affect the whole of Europe within 8 months and subsequently the rest of the world. There is evidence of widespread seeding in Russia and North America during the early months of the pandemic, which was later followed by significant outbreaks. Approximately ten million people worldwide were estimated to be infected by the virus during the pandemic, although the death rate was reported to be relatively low.

1830–1833

The 1830–1833 pandemic started in China in the winter of 1830, and spread rapidly to the Philippines, India and Indonesia, and across Russia into Europe, reaching North America in 1831–1832. The disease re-occurred twice in Europe: in 1831–1832, when the North American outbreak started, and again in 1832–1833. Although this pandemic had a very high attack rate, the mortality rate appears to have been relatively low. As with the 1729–1733 pandemic, there has been discussion about whether this was truly one pandemic or whether the period encompassed multiple events, starting with a period of milder events in 1829–1831 and the true pandemic in 1832–1833.

From 1889 until the 20th century

1889–1892

This pandemic is the first that can truly be described as global, due to the availability of records from across the world. The pandemic started in Russia in May 1889 and was known as Asiatic or Russian influenza. It circulated within Russia until it reached St Petersburg in October 1889. It then continued to spread: Europe and North American ports were affected by the end of the year, and the Mediterranean and North Africa by January 1890. South America, Singapore, India and costal China were affected by February; Australia and New Zealand by March, and sub-Saharan Africa by May 1890. Two further waves of infection occurred in 1891 and 1892 and were probably due to previous seeding. Population attack rates ranged between 25 and 50%, and the number of deaths worldwide was estimated at 300,000. The majority of deaths were in the elderly, and in the later waves.

In Sweden, the Russian flu started spreading in December 1889 and peaked in February 1890, having spread across the country following railway lines and ports, an early indication of the role human travel and transport has played in the spread of influenza. Towns with a railway station or daily sea contact with Stockholm were affected earlier than those that were not transport hubs.

This is the earliest pandemic for which there is serological evidence about the origin of the virus responsible. Studies on serum samples collected before 1957 from people who were alive in 1889 showed A/H2 antibodies, indicating exposure to an A/H2 virus before the 1957 A/H2N2 pandemic began. When A/H2N2 caused the Asian flu pandemic in 1957, the majority of the population had not had previous contact with the virus and so were susceptible; but such prior exposure to an A/H2 virus at the end of the 1800s may explain the relatively lower attack rate in older people.

1898–1900

The origin of this pandemic is not known, but there were large epidemics in Europe, Australia, North America, the Pacific Islands and Japan throughout the period 1898–1900. These outbreaks were mainly mild, and the main interest in this pandemic is serological. Sera collected before 1968 from people alive in 1898 indicate the presence of antibodies to influenza A/H3 and there was lower mortality during the 1968 pandemic in people aged over 75 years, compared with those aged 65–74 years. Again, these people may have had prior exposure to an A/H3 virus at the end of the 19th century.

4.4 Influenza Pandemics of the 20th Century

The following three pandemics (Fig. 4.1) provide much of the knowledge upon which current influenza pandemic preparedness is based; however, despite some similarities in these events, they differed with respect to the causative virus, epidemiology and disease severity, and number of separate waves. Furthermore, there are discrepancies in the literature and reports of differing impacts even within a pandemic both between and within some countries.

1918: Spanish influenza

The Spanish flu pandemic of 1918 coincided with the end of World War I and in a few months was responsible for more deaths than occurred during the preceding 4 years of war. It was caused by an unusually severe strain of influenza A/H1N1. Genetic

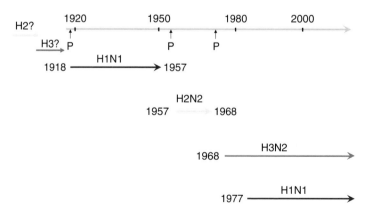

Fig. 4.1. Major influenza A sub-types of the 20th century.

C. Sellwood

sequencing of the virus now suggests this was of avian origin, and that it subsequently adapted to the human host over a period of time prior to the pandemic starting. This may coincide with the somewhat limited evidence of occasional outbreaks of 'severe influenza' in military camps in northern France from 1916 onwards, which may have represented the first incursions into man of an evolving pandemic virus.

The origin of the virus remains unclear; however, it is widely referred to as 'Spanish flu' due to the amount of media reporting and attention the pandemic received in Spain, which was not involved in World War I, compared with the rest of Europe, where wartime news dominated the media. In fact, China and North America have both been identified as possible starting points of the pandemic. In March 1918, three outbreaks were reported simultaneously in the USA (in Detroit, South Carolina and San Quentin Prison) although the virus may have been previously carried to North America from China by labourers, many of whom emigrated from China to the USA at that time. What is known is that from the USA, the pandemic rapidly moved to Europe in early 1918, carried by American troops to France, en route to the battlefields of Western Europe. By April 1918 it had spread across Europe, and had reached epidemic proportions in France. The close confines of military accommodation and the mass deployment and movement of troops involved in World War I may have accelerated initial spread of the pandemic through Europe.

The first report of the pandemic virus in the UK was in Glasgow, Scotland in May 1918, when workers from three factories and an industrial home were taken ill. By June 1918, the virus had been detected in military and naval forces in Portsmouth and other English coastal towns. At the same time, British soldiers in France were becoming infected with the virus, and as they returned to the UK, the troops may have led to the wider infection of the British public. Over the following 6 months the virus spread to North Africa, India, China, New Zealand and the Philippines. Despite extensive quarantine efforts, it finally reached Australia in January 1919.

Many countries experienced second (1918–1919) and third waves (1919–1920) of a more virulent form of infection. The second wave of the pandemic was characterized by three key events where the virus showed increased virulence. An outbreak occurred on a boat travelling from England to Freetown, Sierra Leone. When the boat docked the affected crew were taken to a local hospital and influenza spread among dock workers and local people. It rapidly became clear that the virus was now inflicting a tenfold higher death rate among cases than previously, but this may have been related to underlying susceptibility or nutritional status. At around the same time, a more virulent form of the virus emerged from the port of Brest in France to spread across Europe, and a ship from Europe reached Boston, USA carrying a more virulent form of the virus to seed the disease in North America.

In the UK, the 'Spanish flu' pandemic occurred in three distinct waves. The first occurred in the spring of 1918 and was relatively small. The number of cases reduced, and then peaked again in autumn/early winter 1918, although this time the pattern of infection was very different and the disease much more severe. There was a noticeable increase in clinical attack rate and mortality among adults aged 20–40 years compared with the usual age groups affected by influenza. This became a defining characteristic of the 1918 pandemic, although similar (but less marked) trends towards a relative increase in age-specific mortality in younger adults were also observed in 1957 and 1968. The third wave occurred in early 1919 and was of moderate intensity. Fear of a future 1918-like situation affecting young adults of working age is one particular concern in relation to a future pandemic, although a repeat of such a dramatic shift in age-specific mortality cannot be firmly anticipated.

The severe second wave and moderate third wave occurred during the winter months in the northern hemisphere, which may indicate that pandemic influenza has some association with colder months in line with the recognized seasonality described with seasonal 'interpandemic' influenza (Chapter 1). However, it is recognized that a pandemic can begin at any time of the year – as illustrated by the first wave in spring 1918. In fact, a future 'spring wave' followed by a lull until autumn would 'buy' up to 6 months' time for the production of a pandemic vaccine (Chapter 9).

The reason for the enhanced severity in the second wave, which disproportionately affected young adults, is not known. It is possible that the virus adapted to its new human host between pandemic waves and that the response to infection in young adults involved an intense cytokine response as currently described with human A/H5N1 infections. Older people may have been protected from such an intense response through immune senescence and may have experienced a degree of residual cross-protection due to earlier exposure to a similar virus (possibly in the period prior to the 1889 pandemic). This is discussed later with reference to more recent pandemics. It has also been suggested that the large number of cases in young male adults may have been due in part to the difficult conditions they endured during World War I, which led to increased susceptibility, however, similar mortality rates were observed in civilian females and this theory seems unlikely (Fig. 4.2).

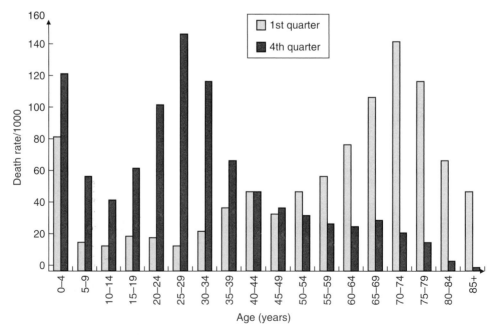

Fig. 4.2. Age-specific influenza death rates among females in England and Wales during the first and fourth quarters of 1918. (Data from HMSO, 1920[1].)

C. Sellwood

Although accurate figures are unavailable in many parts of the world, the pandemic is estimated to have infected 50% of the world's population, half of whom may have suffered a clinically apparent infection. Total excess mortality due to the pandemic is estimated to be at least 40 million although this figure may be quite inaccurate. In the USA more than 600,000 people died and in England and Wales excess civilian deaths numbered about 200,000. Figures 4.3 and 4.4 illustrate the provision of large-scale healthcare in the USA during the 1918 pandemic.

Although the literature is unclear from many developing countries such as India and Africa, there is a general suggestion that case fatality rates were exceptionally high. In some populations, such as in Alaska, southern Africa, India and Western Samoa, extremely high deaths rates were recorded, and in some cases entire villages were reportedly wiped out. In Australia and New Zealand indigenous populations were generally more severely affected than non-native people.

It has been suggested that some of the countries in the southern hemisphere, such as those in South America in which there was relatively little impact from the war, suffered a lower mortality from Spanish flu than countries in the northern hemisphere who were heavily affected by the war. Additionally, the climate and seasons may have had some influence on the number of cases and fatalities; for example, the outbreak in Brazil coincided with the second global wave of the pandemic in October 1918, which was the start of spring in South America, although in the northern hemisphere it was the start of autumn and winter.

The 1918 virus caused the typical clinical symptoms of influenza – acute onset, chills, fever and muscle aches. Bacterial pneumonia reportedly occurred as a complication

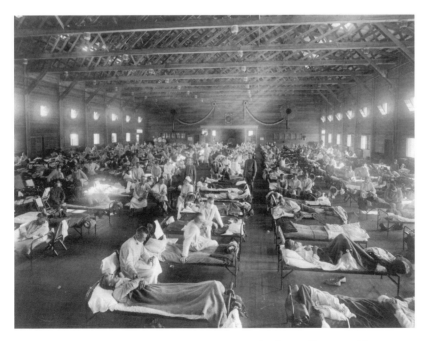

Fig. 4.3. Emergency hospital during the 1918 pandemic, Camp Funston, Kansas. (Photo NCP 1603; courtesy of the National Museum of Health and Medicine, Armed Forces Institute of Pathology, USA.)

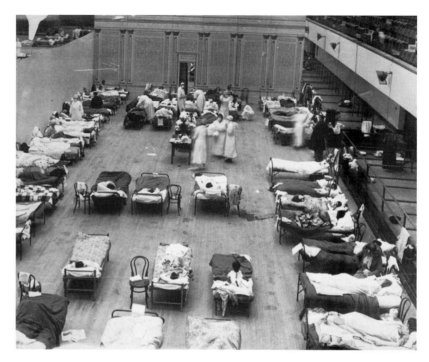

Fig. 4.4. The Oakland Municipal Auditorium in use as a temporary hospital, 1918. (Courtesy of the Oakland Public Library, USA.)

in about 10–15% of cases. In a much smaller proportion of cases the disease was associated with rapid progression and an intense, haemorrhagic, rapidly fatal, viral pneumonitis. Most data sources point to an average case fatality rate of 2.0–2.5%, but in young adults this was around 4%.

The reasons for the very high virulence of this subtype are unknown. Although samples have been recovered from the lungs of victims, including a woman who was recently exhumed from the Alaskan permafrost, there are no definite features of the virus which explain the unusually high mortality. It is now known that the virus was of avian origin but that by 1918 it had definite mammalian characteristics, indicating that for some time prior to the pandemic it may have been circulating in human hosts and slowly adapting through a gradual process of genetic change rather than more abrupt reassortment. In some communities, the pandemic may have been exacerbated by cold weather, lack of heating fuel, overcrowding, mental and physical hardships brought on by the war, and concurrent underlying poor health and malnutrition. There is also evidence that two different strains of the A/H1N1 subtype were co-circulating during the start of the pandemic, with different receptor-binding properties. This may explain the different evolution of the pandemic in different countries.

1957: Asian influenza

The Asian flu pandemic was a global outbreak of avian influenza A/H2N2 that started in Yunnan Province, China in February 1957. Virological evidence indicates that the pandemic virus was a reassorted human and avian influenza virus, a process which probably occurred in an intermediate mammalian host, such as the pig. The haemagluttinin and neuraminidase genes were most likely of avian origin, while the others were derived from the previously circulating A/H1N1 virus.

Within 6 months, the pandemic had spread across the world reaching India, Australia and Indonesia by May; Pakistan, Europe, North America and the Middle East by June; South Africa, South America, New Zealand and the Pacific Islands by July; and Central, West and East Africa, Eastern Europe and the Caribbean by August 1957. Quarantine measures were generally ineffective, and at best merely postponed transmission by a few weeks.

The majority of spread was along shipping lanes, and infections were seen in ports before spreading to urban and rural areas. However, there were two clear overland routes. The first was across Russia to Scandinavia and Eastern Europe as described in earlier events, while the second was less conventional. Almost 2000 delegates from across North America and other countries attended a large conference in Iowa, USA. Many of the delegates were from countries already experiencing epidemics of influenza, and consequently 200 cases occurred during the conference, while many delegates took the infection back home with them when the conference ended.

In Europe the infection was seeded from June 1957 and outbreaks started in September when the autumn school term started. Consequently the illness was first seen in schoolchildren, followed by pre-school children and finally adults. Cases in the UK were concentrated in school-aged children and those crowded together; however, the greatest impact on mortality was in the elderly.

It was thought that the pandemic was over at the end of 1957, but a second wave of infection occurred early in 1958 and affected regions including Europe, North America, Russia and Japan. The two waves were of similar severity in some countries, while in others the second wave caused higher rates of illness and increased fatalities.

The clinical presentation of A/H2N2 in man was rather more typical than in 1918, although high mortality was noted in pregnant women and there was a preponderance of secondary bacterial pneumonia due to *Staphylococcus aureus*. The majority of deaths were in the very young or very old and were due to secondary bacterial pneumonia. The attack rate in older people was lower than in other groups, and may have been due to previous exposure to an influenza A/H2 virus in earlier life. The case fatality rate was less than 0.5% and over one million people died. Although significant, such a level of mortality is several magnitudes lower than is thought to have been the case in 1918.

1968: Hong Kong influenza

The 1968 influenza pandemic also started in China through a process of antigenic reassortment where avian and human viruses combined. The outbreak spread to Hong Kong in July 1968 causing 500,000 cases in just 2 weeks (hence the name 'Hong Kong flu'), from where it rapidly spread to the whole world (Fig. 4.5). However, Japan presents something of a geographical anomaly in that no significant activity due to the new virus was reported until January 1969.

The pandemic reached the USA in September 1968, reportedly via US marines returning to California from Vietnam. By December 1968 the illness was widespread

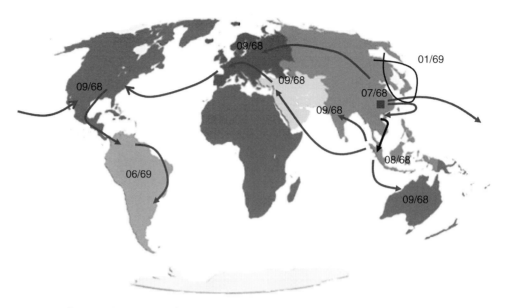

Fig. 4.5. Geographic spread of the 1968–1969 Hong Kong pandemic.

across the USA and morbidity and mortality were as high as in the 1957–1958 pandemic. In Europe the disease was diagnosed from September 1968 onwards; symptoms were mild, excess deaths negligible and demands on medical services were not excessive. However, the number of fatalities due to influenza increased sharply in Europe 1 year later, during the 1969–1970 winter season, and in the UK the epidemic peaked in December 1969. The virus eventually reached South America and South Africa in mid-1969.

In North America, the majority of deaths during this pandemic occurred during the first pandemic wave, while in Europe and Asia the pattern was reversed and the majority of deaths occurred in the second wave. In many countries, local epidemics of the virus were small, causing mild symptoms, and the relative protection of the elderly suggests previous exposure to a similar virus. This theory is supported by serological evidence from samples collected prior to the pandemic from older people who were alive during the 1898–1900 pandemic.

The virus was rapidly identified as influenza A/H3N2 and vaccine manufacture began within 2 months of the virus being isolated. However, only 20 million doses were ready by the time the epidemic peaked in the USA and, because of late deployment, this did not prove a useful control measure.

The 1968–1969 pandemic is estimated to have caused between one to three million fatalities globally – an overall case fatality rate of less than 0.5%. In the UK there were over 30,000 excess deaths attributed to the pandemic, which was no larger than reported for subsequent severe seasonal epidemics in 1976 and 1989.

Thus two of the three pandemics in the last century could be classified as 'mild' compared with 1918. The difference in severity may be explained by the virological origin of each pandemic (Chapter 2). Predicting the severity of a future pandemic is therefore impossible until the virus reveals itself.

C. Sellwood

Focus Box 4.1. Common features of pandemics.

Although the influenza pandemics of the 20th century were not altogether similar, they still have common features that may help indicate what a future pandemic might look like. The available data point to a clinical attack rate that lies in a remarkably narrow range of 25 to 40%. There was more than one pandemic wave in 1918 and in 1968 some countries saw the introduction of the A/H3N2 virus in late winter (January 1969) but experienced the main (second) wave in the following autumn. If one compares the distribution of deaths in 1918 and 1968, it is possible to superimpose both curves in a period lasting about 16 weeks, suggesting that at national level a pandemic wave may last about 4 months from start to finish. Further analyses of existing data have revealed that the impact of a pandemic is likely to be somewhat shorter and sharper at local level (and in closed communities such as prisons) with up to 50% of cases (and the associated deaths and demand for healthcare) occurring in a concentrated 2-week period around the local peak in incidence. In all three pandemics of the 20th century, a shift in age-specific mortality towards younger adults occurred, however, this change was most pronounced in 1918. Most pandemics seem to have originated in Asia, China or Russia. It has been suggested that these geographical areas offer the maximum opportunity for close mixing between man, birds and possibly pigs, allowing more opportunities for genetic reassortment. The interval between pandemics is clearly variable, but looking back far enough, perhaps three such events might be expected each century, giving a crude annualized risk of 3%.

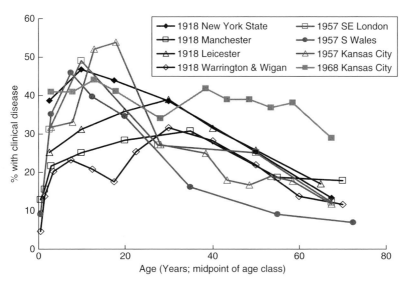

(Reproduced with kind permission of the Modelling and Economics Unit, Health Protection Agency Centre for Infections.)

4.5 Swine Flu, 1976: a Pandemic Averted?

In early 1976, an outbreak of swine influenza (A/H1N1/New Jersey/76) occurred at a US military recruits base in Fort Dix, New Jersey. The outbreak lasted from 19 January until 9 February, and infected at least 230 military personnel, causing 13 hospitalizations for acute respiratory disease and one death. There was great concern that this could herald the start of the next pandemic, especially because it was known that the virus was co-circulating with A/H3N2. A vaccine against swine A/H1N1 was rapidly developed and after a clinical trial of 3000 individuals, a mass vaccination programme of 43 million people was started. However, the association of Guillain–Barré syndrome (a rare neurological condition) with a vaccine made against A/swine/H1N1 led to the premature cessation of the programme. Ultimately no cases of human infection were found outside Fort Dix and this has been a rare instance of an influenza virus with clear human-to-human transmission described, that ultimately failed to spread in the open community. It is not clear whether this was due to the success of the vaccination programme, or the fact that the virus could not spread outside the confines of the recruits' cramped living conditions within the military base.

4.6 Re-emergence of Influenza A/H1N1 in 1977

One year after the swine flu threat, in 1977, human influenza A/H1N1 re-emerged into the human population. The virus did not displace A/H3N2 or cause a pandemic, and has co-circulated with A/H3N2 since its re-emergence. The virus differed genetically from the strain that last circulated prior to the emergence of influenza A/H2N2 in 1957, and instead was more closely related to strains of the virus that circulated during the mid-1940s. Although the re-emergence of A/H1N1 was first reported in Russia in November 1977, it was later determined that is had been present in three Chinese provinces in May 1977. Within 10 months 'Russian flu' (also known as 'red flu') had spread across the globe, via Taiwan, the Philippines, Siberia, Singapore and Russia. By January 1978 it had reached North America, the UK, Central Europe and Japan; by February it had spread to Scandinavia, Southern Europe and the Middle East; and by March to Central America and Australia; finally reaching South America and New Zealand by June 1978. The outbreaks were all mild, and almost all those affected were under the age of 20, who had not been exposed to the virus earlier in their life when it was circulating prior to the 1957 A/H2N2 pandemic. The highest weekly attack rates at the peak of the epidemic reached 13% in children aged 7–14 years.

This event is not described as a true pandemic for a number of reasons. Although it was a global outbreak, it did not infect all age groups; instead the vast majority of cases occurred in people under 20 years of age. The virus closely resembled strains that had circulated previously in human populations. It is unlikely that such a strain could have remained silently in a natural animal or human reservoir, either as a dormant infection or causing undetected cases, without significant antigenic drift occurring such that it was no longer almost identically matched its 1940s progenitor. The resemblance was so great that many feel the re-emergence of this virus was due to a laboratory escape. Lastly, in all previous pandemics for which there are virological

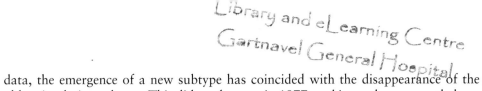
Library and eLearning Centre
Gartnavel General Hospital

data, the emergence of a new subtype has coincided with the disappearance of the older circulating subtype. This did not happen in 1977, and instead we currently have the previously unrecognized situation of two influenza A subtypes co-circulating in human populations: A/H1N1 and A/H3N2.

4.7   Antigenic Recycling in Relation to Human Pandemics

There is strong serological evidence that the pandemics at the end of the 19th century (1889–1891 and 1898–1900) were caused by influenza A/H2 and A/H3, respectively. The three subsequent pandemics of the 20th century were then caused by influenza A/H1N1, A/H2N2 and A/H3N2, and A/H1N1 re-emerged in 1977, to co-circulate with A/H3N2 ever since. This pattern of re-emergence of A/H2, A/H3 and A/H1 viruses in repeated sequence suggests that antigens are recycled and could indicate that these are the only influenza viruses capable of causing widespread human infections and a resultant pandemic.

4.8   Will an Avian Influenza Virus Cause a Future Pandemic?

Avian influenza viruses have the potential to cause disease in man, however, relatively few cases of human disease have been reported due to subtypes other than A/H1, A/H2 and A/H3 – those that have occurred have tended to be either isolated cases or outbreaks of limited size.

Influenza A/H9N2 has caused five known cases of disease in China and Hong Kong since the late 1990s, while A/H7N7 virus caused a large outbreak in the Netherlands in 2003 where 89 people were affected, including one death. Influenza A/H7N3 and A/H7N2 viruses have both caused sporadic disease in the human population, A/H7N3 tending to produce conjunctivitis, while an outbreak of A/H7N2 in the UK in 2007 resulted in three of the four cases being hospitalized on clinical grounds with respiratory symptoms (see Chapter 3).

The avian influenza virus, A/H5N1, is of current concern as having the potential to cause a future pandemic. Avian influenza A/H5N1 first came to prominence in 1997, where an outbreak in Hong Kong poultry led to 18 human cases, of which six were fatal. All poultry in Hong Kong were slaughtered in an attempt to contain the virus, and this was thought to be successful until late 2003, when human cases were identified in China and Vietnam. The virus has been circulating in wild birds and domestic poultry for over a decade in Asia, and has now spread to Africa, Europe and Russia. Since 2003, there have been over 400 human cases of which about 60% have proved fatal. The pattern of disease is severe, with many cases unusually presenting with diarrhoea or multi-organ failure, in addition to the more usual symptoms of influenza. These features have been discussed in greater detail in Chapter 3.

While the current situation with avian influenza A/H5N1 has stimulated the current focus on pandemic preparedness, and the virus is recognized as posing the greatest pandemic threat at the present time, there is still no certainty about which viruses will be responsible for future pandemics.

4.9 Pandemic Preparedness

There is no way at present of predicting the severity of a future pandemic; it may be as globally devastating as the 1918 pandemic, or only slightly worse than a severe seasonal influenza epidemic as in 1968. The northern hemisphere has not experienced a severe winter epidemic since 1989–1990, and while medical facilities continue to improve, many healthcare workers have minimal experience of caring for influenza patients with severe disease. Even fewer of today's healthcare workers were in practice in 1968. Outbreaks of seasonal influenza and instances of increased winter pressures in the health sector due to other viruses or periods of cold weather offer healthcare workers and others the opportunity to exercise pandemic plans, and thus refine preparedness.

The World Health Organization (WHO) has defined a series of six escalating pandemic alert phases to categorize the status of the world regarding a future pandemic (Table 4.2). Global pandemic planning is driven by guidance from WHO, which is supported by national strategic guidance that is operationalized and implemented at the local level. The majority of planning has focused on preparing the health sector to care for an increase in human cases of influenza, however, there is now greater recognition of the need for a whole societal response due to the likely impact of the pandemic across all levels of society (see Chapter 11).

Later chapters focus on the specific impact that previous pandemics have had on different sectors, as well as the impact a future pandemic might have. Pharmaceutical (vaccines, antivirals and antibiotics) and societal interventions (social distancing, public health and infection control measures, and school closures) are discussed, as well as the importance of planning and exercising.

4.10 Summary Points

- The pandemics of the 20th century were caused by three different subtypes of influenza: A/H1N1, A/H2N2 and A/H3N2. They differed in the number of deaths caused and the age groups affected.
- The 1918 pandemic caused by influenza A/H1N1 was the worst pandemic. The pandemic peaked over three waves, with the second wave being the most severe; an estimated 40 million deaths occurred worldwide. Unusually, young adults, aged 20–40 years, were very severely affected by this virus.
- Pandemics have occurred throughout history, and the first recognized pandemic was reported in 1580. Three occurred in the 20th century. There is evidence of antigenic recycling of subtypes A/H1, A/H2 and A/H3.
- Looking back at past pandemics can give an indication of what might be expected, however, nothing is certain. It is impossible to predict the next pandemic virus subtype or its impact.
- The avian influenza A/H5N1 subtype, currently infecting wild birds and domestic poultry across many parts of the world, has been responsible for human cases in Asia, parts of Africa and Europe. Although this virus has been around for over a decade and has not yet acquired the ability for sustained person-to-person spread, it poses a clear pandemic risk.

Table 4.2. World Health Organization (WHO) Revised Pandemic Phases, April 2009 (http://www.who.int/csr/disease/influenza/pipguidance2009/en/index.html).

Phase		
Phase 1	No viruses circulating among animals have been reported to cause infection in people	Predominantly animal infections; few human infections. Pandemic probability uncertain
Phase 2	An animal influenza virus circulating among domesticated or wild animals is known to have caused infection in people and is therefore considered a specific potential pandemic threat	
Phase 3	An animal or human–animal influenza reassortant virus has caused sporadic cases or small clusters of disease in people (e.g. when there is close contact between an infected person and an unprotected caregiver), but has not resulted in human-to-human transmission sufficient to sustain community-level outbreaks	
Phase 4	Human-to-human transmission of an animal or human–animal influenza reassortant virus able to sustain community-level outbreaks has been verified	Sustained human-to-human transmission. Pandemic probability medium to high
Phase 5	The same identified virus has caused sustained community-level outbreaks in two or more countries in one WHO region	Widespread human infection. Pandemic probability high to certain
Phase 6	In addition to the criteria defined in Phase 5, the same virus has caused sustained community-level outbreaks in at least one other country in another WHO region	
Post-peak period	Levels of pandemic influenza activity in most countries with adequate surveillance have declined below peak levels	Possibility of recurrent events
Possible new wave	Levels of pandemic influenza activity in most countries with adequate surveillance are rising again	
Post-pandemic period	Levels of influenza activity have returned to levels seen for seasonal influenza in most countries with adequate surveillance	Disease activity at seasonal levels

Further Reading

Ahmed, R., Oldstone, M.B.A. and Palese, P. (2007) Protective immunity and susceptibility to infectious diseases: lessons from the 1918 influenza pandemic. *Nature Immunology* 8, 1188–1193.

Hsieh, Y.C., Wu, T.Z., Liu, D.P., Shao, P.L., Chang, L.Y., Lu, C.Y., Lee, C.Y., Huang, F.Y. and Huang, L.M. (2006) Influenza pandemics: past, present and future. *Journal of the Formosan Medical Association* 105, 1–6.

Kilbourne, E.D. (2006) Influenza pandemics of the 20th century. *Emerging Infectious Diseases* 12, 9–14.

Morens, D.M. and Fauci, A.S. (2007) The 1918 influenza pandemic: insights for the 21st century. *Journal of Infectious Diseases* 195, 1018–1028.

Potter, C.W. (2001) A history of influenza. *Journal of Applied Microbiology* 91, 572–579.

Viboud, C., Grais, R.F., Lafont, B.A.P., Miller, M.A. and Simonsen, L. (2005) Multinational impact of the 1968 Hong Kong influenza pandemic: evidence for a smouldering pandemic. *Journal of Infectious Diseases* 192, 233–248.

World Health Organization (WHO) (2009) Epidemic and Pandemic Alert and Response (EPR). Pandemic influenza preparedness and response, WHO guidance document. http://www.who.int/csr/disease/influenza/pipguidance2009/en/index.html (accessed April 2009).

Note

[1] Reproduced from an original by J.S. Nguyen-Van-Tam; first appeared in Nguyen-Van-Tam, J.S. (1998) Epidemiology of Influenza. In: Nicholson, K.G., Webster, R.G. and Hay, A.J. (eds) *Textbook of Influenza*. Blackwell Science, Oxford.

C. Sellwood

5 Influenza Transmission and Related Infection Control Issues

J. ENSTONE

- What is known, what can be deduced and what is still unknown about influenza transmission?
- Based on the evidence, what are the most important routes of transmission for influenza?
- What infection control measures can be used to reduce influenza transmission in healthcare settings?
- What measures can be used by the public to reduce influenza transmission?
- Can further research provide better evidence to address the issues still under debate with regard to transmission?

5.1 Introduction

Despite its ubiquitous nature, there is remarkably little influenza-specific evidence in the literature addressing transmission and over the past few years, in the context of pandemic planning, the lack of good evidence has become more apparent. In recognition of this, more research around influenza transmission and the effectiveness of measures to reduce it is now being conducted. The results of some of these studies should soon begin to provide evidence to help better understand the mechanisms of transmission. In the meantime, infection control policies for influenza are based on what we do know about transmission and what can reasonably be deduced. This information comes from a collection of sources including laboratory data, epidemiological studies, outbreak reports and a number of animal and human studies, as well as information on other respiratory viruses.

Clearly, having a good understanding of how influenza is transmitted is critical in order to be able to select the most appropriate and effective non-pharmaceutical interventions and infection control precautions. Furthermore, in a pandemic, supplies of masks and other personal protective equipment (PPE) may run short, so it is important that they are not wasted by being used unnecessarily or inappropriately. Hence there is an urgent need for robust research studies to establish which infection control measures are the most effective in which settings.

Vaccines and antivirals (as prophylaxis or treatment) have an obvious and major role in the prevention and management of seasonal influenza. However, in a pandemic, supplies of appropriate vaccine will initially be limited and antiviral supplies may run short; therefore non-pharmaceutical measures will have a critical role in limiting transmission, especially in resource-poor settings where vaccines and antivirals may prove to be unaffordable.

5.2 What is Known about Influenza Transmission?

Like many infections, influenza is almost certainly transmitted via multiple routes, including by respiratory droplets and contact transmission. Aerosol transmission (via very small particles) may also occur under certain conditions, including during some medical procedures involving the respiratory tract that generate aerosols, but its clinical importance relative to droplet and contact transmission is uncertain and subject to ongoing debate.

Much of what is known about influenza transmission is drawn from relatively old experimental studies and outbreak reports. Over recent years, in the course of pandemic planning, some of these studies have been revisited and it has become increasingly clear that many have confounders and other factors that limit their usefulness. No human-to-human influenza transmission studies have been reported, and although some useful principles can be deduced from work on other respiratory viruses such as respiratory syncytial virus (RSV) and rhinovirus, the results cannot simply be generalized to influenza, as the relative clinical importance of the different modes of transmission varies between organisms.

However, there is more certainty with regard to some aspects of influenza relevant to transmission. It has been shown for influenza that:

- The amount of virus shedding correlates with the severity of symptoms and the presence of fever; this peaks early in the course of the illness.
- Pre-symptomatic and asymptomatic viral shedding also occur.
- Children and the immunocompromised shed virus in higher titres and for longer periods than immunocompetent adults.
- Influenza survives on surfaces for varying amounts of time depending on the type of surface (longer periods on hard non-porous surfaces, shorter periods on porous surfaces), making contact transmission feasible.

5.3 What is Unknown about Influenza Transmission?

Given influenza was first discovered in 1933, there is a surprising amount that is not really understood regarding its transmission. The following are areas where insufficient is known:

- While droplet and contact transmission are generally considered to be the most important routes of transmission for influenza, the relative importance of these is unknown.
- The importance of aerosols in close contact transmission (i.e. within approximately 1 m of an infected individual) is unknown.
- The importance of aerosols in long-distance transmission is unknown.
- It is unclear which medical procedures that generate aerosols are high-risk for influenza transmission.
- The importance of contact transmission is not well understood; it is known that the influenza virus can survive for varied lengths of time depending on the type of surface contaminated, but to date there is no direct evidence that contact with contaminated surfaces results in transmission of infection.

- It is unclear how far respiratory droplets travel before they fall to the ground; some of the evidence from the severe acute respiratory syndrome (SARS) outbreaks in 2003 suggests that droplet transmission occurs beyond the traditional close contact distance of 1 m (a distance based on epidemiological studies of meningococcal disease during the 1980s).
- Although pre-symptomatic and asymptomatic viral shedding are known to occur, their relationship with infectivity is uncertain.
- It is not known whether inoculation with influenza virus via the human eye can cause respiratory infection.
- The relative and incremental benefits of infection control interventions are not known, in particular, no data exist to quantify the relative efficacy of surgical masks compared with respirators in preventing the transmission of influenza.
- The role of simple ventilation measures in reducing transmission is unknown.
- It may be the case that in a pandemic, virus shedding and therefore the period of infectivity will be longer in immunocompetent adults than currently seen with interpandemic (seasonal) influenza, because they are naive to the virus.

5.4 What can Reasonably be Deduced about Influenza Transmission?

Some useful principles can be deduced from work on other respiratory viruses such as RSV and rhinovirus, although the results cannot necessarily be generalized to influenza as the relative clinical importance of the different modes of transmission will vary between organisms; for example, RSV is considered to be transmitted more by contact than droplets so the relative benefits of different infection control interventions will not be the same. On the other hand, hand hygiene has been shown to be effective for several microorganisms and it is reasonable to assume that it will be effective for influenza (if appropriate cleaning agents are used).

In addition to factors that can be deduced from work on other viruses, the following points are reasonable deductions based on what is known about influenza:

- As virus shedding correlates with symptoms, those with asymptomatic infection and those still incubating the disease will be substantially less infectious.
- As immunocompromised people and children shed virus at higher titres and for longer periods than most adults, they will be infectious for a longer period.
- Respiratory secretions play a major part in the transmission of infection, therefore good respiratory hygiene should help reduce (contact and droplet) transmission.
- Regular hand hygiene and environmental cleaning will reduce opportunities for contact transmission as the influenza virus is killed by soap and water and many common household cleaning products.

Evaluating the relative contributions of the different modes of transmission is complex. Proving or ruling out particular modes of transmission is difficult under experimental conditions and significantly harder under natural conditions such as outbreaks, where it is complicated by confounders and the difficulty of distinguishing between the effectiveness of the multiple interventions employed. However, such information would be invaluable for everyday management of respiratory infections, particularly so for a pandemic, so that resources are not wasted where they are not required.

5.5 Modes of Transmission of Infection

Influenza is almost certainly transmitted by more than one route. Traditionally there are three key modes of transmission that have now become common nomenclature in infection control. These are: (i) contact transmission; (ii) droplet transmission; and (iii) airborne transmission. While all are considered relevant to influenza, their relative contribution and importance are not clear.

Contact transmission

Contact transmission can be either direct, which involves organisms being directly transferred from one infected individual to another (susceptible) person, or indirect, which involves transmission via some other contaminated object such as contaminated hands (e.g. hands that have not been properly cleaned after contact with respiratory secretions), tissues or surfaces. The infection is then transmitted by contact with the mucosa, which can be to oneself or to another person.

Droplet transmission

Droplet transmission occurs when respiratory droplets from the respiratory tract of an infected person settle on the mucous membranes of the nose or mouth (or possibly conjunctiva; see below) of another susceptible person. Respiratory droplets are produced by coughing, sneezing and talking, as well as during some medical procedures (e.g. endotracheal intubation). Droplets are generally defined as larger than 5 μm in diameter, but there is no clear consensus about this threshold. Because of their relatively large size, droplets travel only short distances (traditionally a distance of 1 m has been used for infection control purposes, but this is currently subject to debate) before settling on surfaces.

Airborne (or aerosol) transmission

Airborne transmission occurs via aerosolization of microorganisms, including viruses, or the formation of droplet nuclei whereby larger particles dry out to become very small infectious particles. Aerosols are very small particles (typically described as <5 μm in diameter) that can, by virtue of their small size, remain suspended in the air for long periods (at least several hours) and travel over distances far greater than 1–2 m. This allows them to be inhaled by others who may be some distance away from the source. Aerosols can be produced during some medical procedures including endotracheal intubation, manual ventilation and suctioning, cardiopulmonary resuscitation and bronchoscopy, and some of these aerosol-generating procedures (AGPs) might carry an increased risk of disease transmission. Small particles are also present in coughs and

J. Enstone

sneezes but their role in natural influenza infection is uncertain. There is also little evidence of long-distance airborne infection in natural influenza infections (see later).

Conjunctival transmission

There are no reports of human respiratory infection with human influenza solely via conjunctival inoculation, however, it is theoretically possible. The current evidence base to inform advice on the use of goggles for influenza is inadequate and would benefit from further research. Current UK infection control guidance for healthcare workers looking after all patients advises that risk assessments are conducted and where there is thought to be a risk of splashing to the eye, the use of eye protection is recommended. In relation to pandemic influenza, eye protection is advised during AGPs, and other examples might include paediatric nursing care where the patient has poor respiratory etiquette and unusually close or prolonged contact is needed to provide effective care.

5.6   Infection Control Precautions to Counteract Transmission

There are two broad categories into which infection control precautions can be usefully categorized. These are: (i) standard infection control precautions; and (ii) transmission-based precautions.

Standard infection control precautions

Standard infection control precautions (also called 'standard infection control principles' in the UK) were built on the 'universal precautions' introduced during the 1980s by the Centers for Disease Control and Prevention (CDC) in the USA and are intended to reduce the transmission of blood-borne and other nosocomial infections.

Standard precautions should be used for every patient irrespective of infection status (on the principle that some infections, such as blood-borne infections, may not be immediately evident). Standard precautions include hand hygiene, environmental hygiene, the use of PPE, and the safe use and disposal of sharps. More recently in the USA, following the SARS outbreaks, standard precautions have been extended to include respiratory hygiene.

Transmission-based infection control precautions

Based on the three key categories of transmission detailed earlier, there are three categories of transmission-based infection control precautions which are more or less adopted globally by infection control practitioners. These have been devised and refined by CDC, since the late 1970s, and recently updated and expanded in 2007. These categories are: (i) droplet precautions; (ii) contact precautions; and (iii) 'airborne' precautions. Whenever it seems likely that transmission would not be interrupted by standard precautions alone, one or more of the transmission-based precautions should be added.

5.7   Which Infection Control Precautions are Required for Influenza?

Droplet precautions and standard infection control precautions are required for influenza. Although influenza is considered to be transmitted by the contact route as well as the droplet route, it is not necessary to use contact precautions per se because standard infection control precautions already include hand hygiene, cleaning of the environment and the use of PPE. Contact precautions tend to be reserved for circumstances when there are resistant organisms or a more obvious risk from contact, such as when patients have faecal incontinence or significant wound leakage. Standard precautions clearly stipulate the necessity for gloves and PPE when in contact with respiratory secretions. In addition to droplet precautions and standard precautions, good respiratory hygiene should be practised by everyone.

5.8   Counteracting Droplet Transmission

To minimize droplet transmission in the healthcare setting:

- Fluid-repellant surgical masks should be worn when in close contact (i.e. within 1 m) with symptomatic patients (in general, this means putting on a mask when entering a room or cohorted area); in addition to providing a barrier to the nose and mouth, wearing a mask should also help reduce contact transmission as it discourages the wearer from touching their face.
- Ideally, symptomatic patients should be accommodated in single rooms, but these are rare in most healthcare systems and during a pandemic such facilities would be quickly exhausted. Therefore patients should be 'cohorted' (grouped together with other patients who have influenza and no other infection) in a separate area (and cared for by staff who look after only patients with influenza).
- The movement and transport of influenza patients should be kept to an irreducible minimum.
- If transport or movement is necessary, droplet transmission should be reduced by asking patients to wear a surgical mask, but if a mask cannot be tolerated, good respiratory hygiene should be emphasized.

Note that special room ventilation is not considered necessary to counteract droplet transmission.

5.9   Influenza Transmission: the Evidence For and Against the Different Modes of Transmission

Evidence for droplet transmission

The evidence for droplet transmission derives from epidemiological studies of outbreaks. When used alongside other interventions such as hand hygiene, the addition of precautions against droplet transmission appears to contain outbreaks of influenza. Outbreak reports from a variety of settings including a hospital ward (where staff and patients became ill and patterns of spread suggested staff were responsible for disseminating influenza to 24 other patients on the ward) and a correctional facility (where all cases were in single rooms and all new cases had contact with known cases) displayed time and place characteristics suggestive of close contact transmission, which could have been via either droplet or contact.

Evidence for contact transmission

Influenza virus has been shown to survive on hard non-porous surfaces (in one commonly cited study, these were a stainless steel counter and a plastic washing-up bowl) for up to 72 h, although little was detected beyond 48 h. In contrast, virus was recovered from soft porous items (e.g. cotton and paper items) for only up to 24 h, and only small quantities after 12 h.

In the same study the transferability of influenza A virus from contaminated surfaces on to hands was also evaluated. The results suggest that people shedding large amounts of virus can transmit via stainless steel surfaces for between 2 and 8 h and via paper tissues for a few minutes. In this particular study, virus survived for only 5 min on hands – but theoretically long enough for onward transmission to either oneself or others through touch or contamination of other objects.

In a different study, influenza virus was recovered from objects in a nursery where children had influenza, and virus was also found on more than half of the objects swabbed in the children's homes. However, no studies have been published that prove that influenza infection has resulted from contact with contaminated objects or contaminated hands; but this has not been adequately ruled out either.

Contaminated hands undoubtedly play a part in the transfer of infection. Studies have documented caregivers' hands becoming contaminated after activities involving infected patients. This has been shown for a multitude of bacteria and RSV although no studies have specifically looked at influenza. Other studies have shown cross-contamination by hands, including viruses, but again these were not influenza-specific.

Observational studies have also indicated contact transmission. One outbreak report from a neonatal unit found an association between twin births and mechanical ventilation and acquiring influenza. It was hypothesized that parents handling their twins without washing their hands between was responsible for the association. It was also hypothesized that babies on mechanical ventilation might also have required extra handling, in addition to the ventilator tubing being a possible route of infection.

Evidence for aerosol or airborne transmission

Limited data are available to evaluate the role of aerosol or airborne transmission in man. Experimental infection by inhalation of aerosolized virus has been shown to induce symptomatic illness more readily than the instillation of nasal drops (i.e. droplets) and at lower doses, but how well this represents natural transmission is not certain.

Some observational studies purport to support aerosol transmission but the evidence is not necessarily very convincing. One report cited as evidence of aerosol transmission dates from the 1957 influenza pandemic. There was less influenza among tuberculosis patients in a ward where there was ultraviolet (UV) lighting (2% of patients, compared with almost 20% of patients in a non-radiated ward), which might suggest that the UV radiation had inactivated viral-containing aerosols (the UV radiation was positioned such that it reached only the upper air in the room where aerosols would be present; in addition, UV is not effective for surface decontamination because of poor penetration and not effective for droplets because the humidity of droplets is too high for UV to be effective). However, the two wards were in different buildings and there is no evidence that the exposure to influenza was the same in both wards.

In another observational study, published in 1979 and often cited as evidence for airborne transmission, a high proportion of crew and passengers developed an influenza-like illness within 72 h of being on a plane with a passenger with influenza symptoms. The flight was delayed for a number of hours on the ground in Alaska, with the ventilation system turned off. Although the high attack rate and the fact that even passengers at some distance from the source were infected might be suggestive of airborne infection, transmission by droplet or contact spread cannot be ruled out as passengers moved freely about the plane while it was on the tarmac.

Some animal studies suggest a role for aerosol transmission. However, the results of such studies need to be interpreted with care when generalizing them to human transmission as it is difficult to model human influenza in animals, where transmission mechanisms might not be identical. Some old studies using mice have given some support to aerosol transmission. In one study mice became infected up to 24 h after influenza virus was aerosolized in a room, although the proportion infected decreased over time. However, mice have since been shown to be a less than ideal model for transmission per se as human influenza does not transmit well from mouse to mouse. More recently animal studies using guinea pigs and ferrets have been favoured. Ferrets share the same receptors in respiratory epithelial cells as found in the human respiratory tract, so are potentially a better model for transmission than mice. They also manifest similar influenza symptoms to human subjects, but are large, can be difficult to handle and are expensive. Because of these disadvantages, the guinea pig, where droplet transmission has been proved, has been identified as a useful alternative model for transmission studies.

Despite the difficulties in mimicking human transmission in animals, animal models have potential to help define parameters for human studies particularly as they become more sophisticated. In addition, exploration of the virological and physiological issues of influenza transmission – or the lack of it – in animal models may cast a useful light on possible reasons why, for example, people do not easily acquire or transmit avian influenza virus infection.

The dynamics of and particle size composition of coughs and sneezes are not very clear and will vary significantly from person to person. Coughs and sneezes are made up of particles of varying sizes and there is unlikely to be a precise size cut-off where transmission changes from droplet to aerosol. So, while coughs and sneezes are likely to contain mainly droplets they will also contain a proportion of aerosol-sized particles, and the relative importance of droplets and aerosols in transmission is not known.

J. Enstone

5.10 The Debate: Current Thinking Regarding Influenza Transmission

Influenza transmission almost certainly occurs through multiple routes and although there is no evidence that establishes which of these modes of transmission is the most important, epidemiological patterns of influenza in hospital, nursing homes, community settings and observational studies frequently support close-range transmission, suggesting that droplet and contact transmission are likely to be the most significant routes. This is not to say that airborne/aerosol transmission does not occur, but convincing evidence of airborne transmission between people over long distances is lacking. However, the paucity of evidence for transmission over long distances does not rule out aerosols being infectious at a closer distance, such as aerosols generated by some medical procedures, or from the smaller particles in coughs and sneezes. The importance of these small particles in natural influenza transmission is not known. Although coughs and sneezes are made up predominantly of droplets that are too large to become airborne, a single sneeze supposedly contains a sufficient proportion of aerosol-sized particles to be significantly infectious; however, this theoretical risk is not that well substantiated by real-life examples, especially regarding spread over longer distances. Despite this theoretical infectiousness, the reproductive number (R_0) for influenza is relatively low (usually less than 2) even when pre-existing immunity is low; this value of R_0 is not consistent with a highly infectious organism such as measles virus. So clearly there are still elements of influenza transmission that remain poorly understood.

It has been argued that the importance of airborne transmission might be played down by some investigators due to an unwillingness to acknowledge its importance, perhaps because of the potential economic impact and practical difficulties of implementing airborne precautions, such as special ventilation and the expense and training required if respirators need to be the respiratory protection of choice during a pandemic.

There is also international debate about the maximum distance over which droplet transmission is thought to occur. Since the SARS outbreaks in 2003 there has been debate about whether the distance that droplets might travel may be closer to 2–3 m rather than 1 m, and certainly in the USA, the advice is to treat the traditionally accepted 1 m as an approximation of what is meant by close distance and not treat it as a precise cut-off point. Currently there is no consensus on this, either between countries or between institutions. Definitive studies could usefully be performed to give a robust answer to this question.

5.11 Counteracting Transmission

Counteracting droplet and contact transmission

Surgical masks

Surgical face masks were initially introduced to be worn by those in close proximity to patients during surgery to help maintain a sterile field. However, their use to protect healthcare workers from infected patients is also longstanding, dating from the time of the 1918 pandemic. Nowadays surgical masks have three main purposes:

(i) to protect the patient during 'sterile' procedures; (ii) to protect healthcare workers and others from respiratory secretions or other splashes by acting as a fluid-resistant physical barrier to the nose and mouth; and (iii) to limit the spread of infection from coughing and sneezing patients to others. When worn by a healthcare worker, as well as acting as a barrier, a mask will also act as good reminder to avoid touching the face. Masks should not be touched on the outside by the wearer after exposure to an influenza patient as hands could easily become contaminated which could result in onwards transmission, to oneself, to others or to some inanimate object.

Reports following the SARS epidemic indicated that surgical masks provided healthcare workers with some protection when in close contact with patients. One case–control study looked at the PPE reported as being used by staff both infected and not infected with SARS following exposure to patients with SARS. The findings were that a face mask was significantly protective against the transmission of SARS. But as in any case–control study, recall bias cannot be entirely excluded. The second study was a cohort study in Toronto, again looking at PPE used in different situations. This study concluded that wearing a mask or N95 respirator (similar to FFP2) offered significant protection, but the numbers were too small to allow separate conclusions to be drawn regarding surgical face masks and respirators, or explore possible differences in protection between the two interventions.

The lack of conclusive evidence for or against the effectiveness of face masks in preventing influenza transmission has led to a number of recent randomized trials to determine the effectiveness of face masks in community settings. From the studies that have been published to date (only a minority), a protective effect of mask wearing against influenza transmission has not been so far demonstrated. This is in part due to the difficulties in such community studies of poor compliance with mask wearing and other interventions. However, in one study, a secondary analysis showed that full compliance with mask wearing resulted in a relative reduction in the daily risk of acquiring a respiratory infection by 60–80%. This study used a clinical definition of influenza-like illness or laboratory confirmation of one or more respiratory viruses as outcomes. In reality relatively few cases of influenza were diagnosed, in fact more cases of rhinovirus were confirmed than influenza. Thus the findings of the study are not easily applied to influenza because the relative importance of different modes of transmission almost certainly varies between different pathogens. Thus, at the present time, the available new evidence does not change the situation regarding the uncertainty of the effectiveness of face masks against human influenza – although they are still not proved to be effective, neither are they proved to be ineffective.

Distancing

Traditionally, based on epidemiological evidence regarding meningococcal disease, the area of risk for droplet transmission has been considered to be 1 m around the infected patient and, historically, putting on masks at this distance has been effective in preventing infections thought to be spread by droplets. However, CDC isolation guidance was updated in 2007 to suggest that this distance should be used as an approximation rather than an absolute distance. As well as 1 m being the distance used to advise healthcare workers when to put on face masks, it is also the recommended distance for bed separation in healthcare settings.

J. Enstone

Personal protective equipment

PPE includes disposable gloves and plastic aprons, gowns and eye protection to protect the wearer. Plastic aprons protect clothing and should be changed between patients and gloves help prevent contact transmission between patients or to the wearer. They must also be changed between patients and between different tasks on the same patient. It should be noted that glove wearing is not a substitute for hand hygiene.

Different PPE should be used depending upon the activity being undertaken. Table 5.1 shows the PPE advised in the UK for various levels of patient contact when working in healthcare settings during a pandemic.

Under standard infection control precautions eye protection or face shields should be worn when there is a risk of splashes to the eye. However, it is not known whether inoculation with influenza virus solely via the eye can cause respiratory infection. Current UK pandemic infection control guidance advises that a risk assessment is carried out to decide whether to use eye protection or a face shield, except during AGPs when this is always recommended. Further research on conjunctival inoculation would help inform guidance on this issue.

Environmental cleaning

Data demonstrating the effectiveness of environmental cleaning in reducing transmission of influenza are very limited, but given that the influenza virus is killed by soap

Table 5.1. Personal protective equipment for care of patients in a healthcare setting with pandemic influenza. (Reproduced from *Pandemic Influenza: Guidance for Infection Control in Hospital and Primary Care Settings*, 2007, by kind permission of the Department of Health, England.)

	Entry to cohorted area but no patient contact	Close patient contact (within 1 m)	Aerosol-generating procedures[a]
Hand hygiene	✓	✓	✓
Gloves	✗[b]	✓[c]	✓
Plastic apron	✗[b]	✓	✗
Gown	✗	✗[d,e]	✓[e]
Surgical mask	✓[f]	✓	✗
FFP3 respirator	✗	✗	✓
Eye protection	✗	Risk assessment	✓

[a]Wherever possible, aerosol-generating procedures should be performed in side rooms or other closed single-patient areas with minimal staff present.
[b]Gloves and apron should be worn during cleaning procedures.
[c]Gloves should be worn in accordance with standard infection control precautions. If glove supplies become limited, glove use should be prioritized for contact with blood and body fluids, invasive procedures, and contact with sterile sites.
[d]Consider in place of apron if extensive soiling of clothing or contact of skin with blood and other body fluids is anticipated (e.g. during intubation or caring for babies).
[e]If a non-fluid-repellent gown is used, a plastic apron should be worn underneath.
[f]Surgical masks (fluid-repellent) are recommended for use at all times in cohorted areas for practical purposes. If mask supplies become limited or pressurized, then in cohorted areas use should be limited to close contact with a symptomatic patient (within 1 m).

and water, detergent and other household cleaning agents, cleaning will reduce transmission. Therefore frequently touched surfaces and objects should be cleaned regularly – twice daily is suggested for patient areas. Household detergent is perfectly adequate to kill influenza; disinfectants are not necessary, and in the healthcare environment, actively discouraged unless they are required for gastrointestinal outbreaks such as *Clostridium difficile* or norovirus. In healthcare settings, gloves, plastic aprons and surgical masks should be worn when cleaning in areas where there are infected patients.

Hand hygiene

Hand hygiene is one of the main elements of standard infection control precautions. UK guidelines for preventing healthcare-associated infections indicate that effective hand decontamination markedly reduces the carriage of pathogens on the hands and so it follows that hand hygiene will decrease the transmission of influenza by the contact route.

Hand hygiene has been shown to be particularly effective in young children in reducing respiratory virus infections, and has also been shown to reduce mortality from respiratory disease. However, no hand hygiene studies specific to influenza have been published.

Hands should be cleaned after patient contact, or contact with the patient's environment, with either soap and water or an alcohol hand rub.

Respiratory hygiene

Respiratory hygiene includes using disposable tissues for covering coughs and sneezes and for wiping runny noses. Used tissues should be binned or flushed away immediately and then hands should be cleaned. Studies show that the use of antiviral tissues (where the antiviral agents included citric acid) is effective in reducing contact transmission of 'colds' due to rhinovirus infection when compared with normal cotton handkerchiefs.

Counteracting aerosol transmission

Respirators are designed to protect the wearer from airborne particles and aerosols. They have a higher filtering specification than surgical masks and should be used in healthcare settings in circumstances where there is a high risk of exposure to aerosols which carry an increased risk of transmission. Uncertainty about the mode of transmission of influenza influences the debate about whether it might be appropriate to use respirators for all close patient contact, instead of surgical masks.

Respirators are categorized according to their filtering efficiency and are made to specific standards. The European standard EN149:2001 covers Filtering Face Piece 1 (FFP1), FFP2 and FFP3 respirators. FFP3 respirators have the highest filtering efficiency and are broadly similar but not identical to the N99 respirator, which is made to a US standard. The next highest filtering respirator available is the FFP2, which is broadly similar but not identical to the US N95 respirator. Respirators need to be fit-tested for every individual and then fit-checked with each wearing to be effective. They are not effective if not fitted correctly, i.e. achieving a good seal around the nose and mouth; this makes them particularly unsuitable for use by the public and untrained healthcare workers.

Most respirators are designed to be single-use only. They are many times more expensive than surgical masks and are harder to use correctly because they need fit-testing. They can also be uncomfortable if worn for long periods and have been reported as making the performance of some tasks more difficult and slower than usual. All of these factors will influence any policy decision about recommending them for widespread use during a pandemic, as incorrect use would significantly compromise their effectiveness. Interestingly, a meta-analysis of the SARS outbreak data found limited evidence of the incremental effectiveness of respirators over surgical masks.

5.12 Aerosol-generating Procedures

In the UK, FFP3 respirators are recommended for use when there is exposure to aerosols, such as those generated during some medical procedures, which may carry an increased risk of infection. However, there is uncertainty and debate over when the risk of influenza transmission from aerosols may be high. Some aerosol-generating procedures (AGPs) have been associated with an 'increased risk of disease transmission'. Adapted from a list of procedures published by the World Health Organization (WHO) in 2007, the procedures considered to be associated with an increased risk of disease transmission are intubation and related procedures (e.g. manual ventilation and suctioning), cardiopulmonary resuscitation and bronchoscopy. Although none of these procedures has had this risk specifically evaluated for influenza, in the absence of evidence specific to influenza, UK pandemic infection control guidance advises that healthcare workers use an FFP3 respirator in rooms when such procedures are carried out.

There are also additional procedures that have been categorized by WHO as procedures with a 'controversial/possible' increase in risk of respiratory pathogen transmission, which are procedures that only may be associated with an increased risk. The procedures in this category are non-invasive positive pressure ventilation, high-frequency oscillating ventilation and nebulization.

Because the risk of influenza transmission is currently uncertain for these 'controversial/possible' procedures, current UK infection control advice takes a cautious approach and advises that an FFP3 respirator is also used for these AGPs until a more detailed assessment of risk with regard to influenza has been made. Inevitably this means that further research is needed.

During procedures likely to generate aerosols, only essential healthcare workers should be present in the immediate vicinity, and if at all possible AGPs should be carried out in single rooms with the doors shut. In addition to respirators, gowns, eye protection and gloves should be worn (see Table 5.1).

5.13   Translating Evidence on Transmission into Practical Advice

Practical infection control advice for healthcare settings

A variety of measures can be used to reduce the risk of transmission of influenza in the healthcare setting. These are put in place to reduce transmission between patients, from patient to healthcare worker, and from healthcare worker to patient.

It should be borne in mind that although healthcare workers are at risk from patients in healthcare facilities with influenza, they are also likely to be in contact with influenza in the community outside working hours, and are arguably at greater risk of being exposed to infection there. If healthcare workers do feel ill with symptoms of influenza it is important that they do not come to work.

Some of the measures are administrative and include separating patients with and without influenza and having separate staff caring for each group. This can be achieved in different ways depending upon the setting. For example, patients on a hospital ward or in a nursing home can be cohorted and looked after by staff who do not move between them and patients without influenza; in primary care settings, a waiting area can be split so that patients with respiratory symptoms do not mix with patients without respiratory symptoms. Patients can be asked to wear a surgical mask when in communal areas or when moving from one area to another, to help reduce transmission.

In brief, reducing the transmission of influenza in the healthcare setting involves:

- Instructing staff with respiratory symptoms to stay at home.
- Segregating patients with influenza as soon as possible.
- Separating staff into those who deal with influenza patients and those who do not.
- Restricting access for visitors who are symptomatic.
- Implementing standard and droplet precautions including surgical mask use, good hand hygiene and the correct use of PPE according to risk of exposure (see Table 5.1), which includes removing and disposing of it carefully (as clinical waste) to prevent contamination.
- Frequent environmental cleaning with water and detergent or detergent wipes (twice daily in clinical areas).
- Encouraging good respiratory hygiene – tissues and access to bins should be provided.

Infection control advice for public settings and the family home

The results of community studies looking at various interventions (such as hand hygiene and mask wearing) to reduce the transmission of influenza and other acute respiratory infections, often suggest that the public are poor at complying with infection control advice. It may be that, in the event of a pandemic, compliance is improved due to the fear factor, which is impossible to mimic during research studies. However, advice for the use in the family home during a pandemic needs to be simple and pragmatic to increase the likelihood of compliance.

J. Enstone

In the UK National Framework for Responding to an Influenza Pandemic and Supporting Guidance, advice is provided on infection control and personal hygiene for the public. In brief, anyone ill with influenza-like symptoms should stay at home, minimize social/family contact and go out only if absolutely necessary until their symptoms have resolved. It is also advised that those without influenza can reduce their risk of catching it by avoiding unnecessary close contact with others and by adopting high standards of hygiene including hand hygiene, respiratory hygiene and cleaning in the home.

In principle, the infection control advice for public settings is very similar to that for healthcare facilities. The public should:

- Stay at home when ill with influenza-like symptoms.
- Isolate anyone who is ill (as far as is practical) and if possible nominate one adult family member as the caregiver.
- Use tissues when coughing and sneezing and dispose of them promptly – flushing them away or putting them in a bin or bag.
- Whether symptomatic or not, wash hands frequently with soap and water, which will reduce the chances of picking up the virus from surfaces and reduce its spread from the hands to the face or to other people; this should be done particularly after blowing the nose or disposing of tissues.
- Clean frequently touched hard surfaces (e.g. kitchen worktops, door handles) often, using normal household cleaning products.
- Avoid crowded gatherings where possible, especially in enclosed spaces.
- For cases only (not other family members), wear a disposable mask to protect others should it become absolutely essential to go out while symptomatic.

There is little evidence that generalized widespread use of masks by the public would be useful and therefore most authorities do not advocate stockpiling masks for general use; a far more important recommendation is that symptomatic people should stay at home. However, it is not unreasonable for a household member who is acting as the caregiver to a relative or friend who is ill with pandemic influenza (in effect acting as a lay health attendant) to wear a disposable face mask when in close contact (in the same room) as the patient. In addition, masks may be considered in specific occupational settings after a thorough risk assessment.

5.14   Unresolved Questions for Further Research

The evidence base for both how influenza is transmitted, and for the effectiveness of interventions to reduce it, is poor. There are a number of important research gaps that would benefit from further research, as follows:

1. What is the relative importance of droplet, contact and aerosol transmission?
2. How important are pre-symptomatic and asymptomatic transmission (and how might they occur)?
3. Which AGPs carry a significant risk of transmission for influenza?
4. How important is aerosol transmission outside of AGPs?
5. What is the effectiveness and efficacy of surgical masks and how does this compare with respirators?

6. Can touching surfaces contaminated with influenza virus cause influenza infection?
7. Does ventilation (including simple measures such as opening windows) have a role in reducing transmission?
8. What distance defines 'close contact', i.e. how far do respiratory droplets travel?
9. Can inoculation via the conjunctival mucosa cause respiratory infection?
10. Can masks and respirators be safely decontaminated for re-use?

5.15 Summary Points

- We know that virus shedding correlates with severity of symptoms and that the duration of shedding can vary according to age and immune status. We also know that the virus can survive for varying amounts of time on different surfaces. We can deduce that transmission is likely to be less (but not non-existent) during the incubation period and from asymptomatic individuals. We can also assume that hand hygiene, environmental cleaning and good respiratory hygiene will help reduce transmission. We do not know the relative importance of droplet, contact and airborne (or aerosol) transmission, nor the relative effectiveness or efficacy of most infection control measures.
- Based on epidemiological and observational evidence the most important routes of transmission for influenza are droplet and contact transmission.
- In healthcare settings, in addition to standard infection control precautions (which should be used for all patients irrespective of infection status), precautions against respiratory droplets should be used for patients with confirmed or suspected pandemic influenza. Together these infection control precautions involve good hand and respiratory hygiene, separating patients with influenza from those without influenza, cleaning frequently touched surfaces regularly, and wearing a surgical mask, gloves and plastic aprons for close patient contact. Additional precautions including FFP3 respirators are required for procedures that generate aerosols.
- The public should stay at home if ill and clean their hands and frequently touched surfaces well and often. Care should also be taken to use tissues when coughing, sneezing or wiping the nose. Contact with those who are ill should be minimized where possible.
- Debates continue regarding the occurrence and importance of airborne or aerosol transmission (relative to droplet and contact transmission) both during natural transmission and during the performance of AGPs, where evidence is lacking about which procedures carry an increased risk of transmission. Debate is also ongoing around the distance to which respiratory droplets can travel. These debates, and the debate around masks versus respirators, continue because of the major implications for policy. Well-designed research could provide better and stronger evidence to clarify the issues and resolve the debates.

Further Reading

Bean, B., Moore, B.M., Sterner, B., Petersen, L.R., Gerding, D.N. and Balfour, H.H. Jr (1982) Survival of influenza viruses on environmental surfaces. *Journal of Infectious Diseases* 146, 47–51.

Brankston, G., Gitterman, L., Hirji, Z., Lemieux, C. and Gardam, M. (2007) Transmission of influenza A in human beings. *Lancet Infectious Diseases* 7, 257–265.

Bridges, C.B., Kuehnert, K.J. and Hall, C.B. (2003) Transmission of influenza: implications for control in hospital settings. *Clinical Infectious Diseases* 37, 1094–1101.

Centers for Disease Control and Prevention (2007) *Guideline for Isolation Precautions: Preventing Transmission of Infectious Agents in Healthcare Settings 2007.* http://www.cdc.gov/ncidod/dhqp/gl_isolation.html (accessed May 2009).

Department of Health (2007) *Pandemic influenza: guidance for infection control in hospitals and primary care settings.* http://www.dh.gov.uk/en/Publicationsandstatistics/Publications/PublicationsPolicyAndGuidance/DH_080771 (accessed May 2009).

MacIntyre, C.R., Cauchemez, S., Dwyer, D.E., Seale, H., Cheung, P., Browne, G., Fasher, M., Wood, J., Gao, Z., Booy, R. and Ferguson, N. (2009) Face mask use and control of respiratory virus transmission in households. *Emerging Infectious Diseases* 15, 233–241.

World Health Organization (2007) *Infection prevention and control of epidemic- and pandemic-prone acute respiratory diseases in health care.* http://www.who.int/csr/resources/publications/WHO_CD_EPR_2007_6/en/index.html (accessed May 2009).

6 The Role of Emergency Planning, Business Continuity and Exercises in Pandemic Preparedness

J. Simpson and C. Sellwood

- How does pandemic influenza preparedness differ from more standard emergency preparedness?
- What is the role of business continuity planning in pandemic preparedness?
- Why is it important that health sector pandemic influenza exercises involve partner organizations?
- Why is time a problem in the design of pandemic influenza exercises?
- Why has the development of 'off-the-shelf' exercises been important in pandemic influenza preparedness?

6.1 Introduction

By its very nature, an influenza pandemic is a global event that will ultimately affect almost every country in the world and almost every community within affected countries. Global preparedness is led by the World Health Organization (WHO) with other bodies, such as the European Centre for Disease Prevention and Control and the United Nations Pandemic Influenza Contingency, interpreting such international guidance to reflect specific challenges. Nevertheless, international plans can only address the broadest principles and strategic issues, and provide technical assistance on specific subjects. It is the role of policy makers and planners at national, regional and local levels within countries to consider what the issues will be for communities and individuals on the ground, and how these can be managed or mitigated.

Countries across the world are working on all aspects of pandemic preparedness (see regional case studies, Chapters 14–16). Much of this has focused on health planning, but as time has passed there has been a greater recognition of the need for a whole-of-society response (Chapter 11). One of the key aspects of pandemic planning is how to deal with the first few cases in a country or city (Case Study 1, Chapter 14). While the 1968 pandemic took around 2–4 months to travel from its point of origin in South-east Asia to the rest of the world, it is anticipated that global spread will be much quicker when the next pandemic occurs. All major air hubs are at most 72 h apart, and it can be predicted that a virus originating in South-east Asia could reach Europe within 2–4 weeks.

It is essential that countries and individual organizations prepare in advance for a pandemic, and that those plans are refined through a process of exercising and testing. This chapter considers the basics of emergency preparedness and business continuity planning (BCP), as well as the importance of exercises in pandemic preparedness.

©CAB International 2010. *Introduction to Pandemic Influenza*
(eds J.S. Nguyen-Van-Tam and C. Sellwood)

6.2 Emergency Preparedness and Business Continuity Planning

In the light of disasters that have occurred in recent years, such as the 9/11 terror attacks on the World Trade Center in 2001, the 2004 tsunami and Hurricane Katrina in 2005 (Chapter 11), and also realization that a future influenza pandemic is inevitable, there has been renewed emphasis on the need for robust emergency preparedness and BCP. Adequate planning and preparation are resource-intensive, time-consuming activities. As a consequence it can be difficult to persuade key decision makers to invest sufficiently, particularly when there are often other pressing needs that require funding now. In some instances this can lead to organizations undertaking the easy parts of emergency planning, such as producing policy and strategy documents, with rather less work directed towards 'translational preparation'.

In this context, translational preparation means turning all the theoretical planning into reality, and practising the responses with appropriate personnel and other resources. Unfortunately, this work is particularly expensive and time-consuming and it can be difficult to persuade the senior members of governments and organizations to engage when the threat is perceived to be distant or abstract. For all these reasons, it is vital that preparation and preparedness is led by individuals or teams with sufficient stature and robustness to garner the support of the organization. This can be a problem if the functions are devolved to junior members of the organization, which is a situation not unfamiliar to some in the emergency planning profession.

Business continuity planning

As planning continues and there is greater awareness of the likely scale and impact of a pandemic on all sectors of society, pandemic preparedness is now a feature of many organizations' business continuity plans to ensure they can continue to function during a pandemic.

A pandemic is a different sort of emergency from those that most organizations are used to planning for: it is a 'rising tide' scenario (gradual onset – long duration) rather than 'big bang' (sudden onset – short duration). Organizations are generally well versed in planning for and responding to a 'big bang' event such as a bomb or flood, which is usually a localized event that occurs rapidly and with little or no warning. Businesses could face reduced staff numbers, interruptions to supplies and disruption to telecommunications, but aid and assistance are usually available from unaffected areas outside the flood or unaffected by the bomb. In addition, the acute phase of the incident is usually over in less than 7 days. In contrast, during a pandemic, all areas will be affected and the scope for mutual aid will be limited; the acute incident will build slowly and last several weeks. In a pandemic, the major impact will be on staff, rather than on information technology infrastructure or buildings, however, there are likely to be knock-on effects to other areas such as supplies, transport, food, fuel and utilities as staff in these sectors become unwell.

BCP requires the essential parts of an organization (e.g. products, staff, buildings) to be identified, and that plans be put in place to ensure these can be maintained if an incident occurs that could cause major disruption to the organization. The key stages involve identifying:

- The organization's key products and services.
- The critical activities and resources required to deliver the key products/services.
- The risks to the critical activities.
- How to maintain the critical activities in the event of a disruption.

Planning and management of business continuity in any organization requires support from senior management from the outset, and one or more nominated individuals to drive things forward and ensure the process is completed and managed through exercising, reviewing and updating plans.

Business impact assessment

The business impact analysis process identifies and documents the key products and services of a business. It then identifies the critical activities needed to deliver these, the impact a disruption would have on them (for the first 24 h, 24–48 h, up to 1 week and up to several weeks) and the resources needed to bring them back on line (Table 6.1). The process helps organizations to identify the maximum length of time a business could cope with disruptions without being overwhelmed or damaged significantly.

Risk assessment

The risk assessment looks at the likelihood and impact of a range of scenarios or risks that could interrupt a business. This is followed by prioritizing those risks and considering the potential consequences of the risks, identifying actions to take and prioritizing those actions.

Typical risk scenarios are: damage or denial of access to premises, loss or damage to information/communication technology, non-availability of key staff, loss or damage to other key resources (e.g. utilities), loss of key partners/resources, disruption to transport. For each scenario, the likelihood of it happening and impact if it did happen should be ranked from high to low (Fig. 6.1). The overall risk is then determined by multiplying the two together. Each risk can then be allocated an action level: reduce, manage or tolerate.

Scenarios that require planning and/or reduction are taken forward to the next stage of the business continuity process, while scenarios that require management and/or can be tolerated can be considered outside the business continuity process.

Table 6.1. Key considerations for the business impact assessment.

Identify key products/services	Those that will have the greatest impact if disrupted
Identify the impact a disruption would have	For the first 24 h, 24–48 h, up to 1 week, up to 2 weeks, longer
Identify critical activities	By considering key products/services and impact
Identify resources needed to bring things back on line	Consider people (ideal and minimum staffing numbers, skill level needed), premises (standard and alternative locations, equipment), technology (computers, telephones), information (market knowledge) and partners (who are your current/alternative suppliers/tenderers)

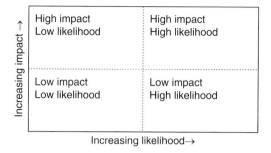

Fig. 6.1. The risk assessment matrix.

The business continuity plan

The final stage of the process is to assemble all the available information and produce a strategy that details how services will be maintained in the event of a disruption, covering risk reduction and recovery measures. Some parts of the overall strategy could be proactive (e.g. a cost-effective intervention applied before the scenario occurs in order to mitigate the subsequent effect of the incident), while others will be reactive, ready to be implemented when the scenario occurs. These form the basis of the business continuity plan. Issues that cannot be addressed through BCP still need addressing elsewhere within the organization.

6.3   Interdependency and Interoperability

It is essential that interdependencies are considered in the BCP process, otherwise there is a risk for example that all businesses will assume the same alternative venue is available. Additionally, business continuity plans must be considered as 'living documents', and they should be exercised and tested regularly, with updates to reflect new guidance or lessons learned. Staff should be familiar with the business continuity plan before it is needed; there will not be time in the middle of an incident to pull the plan off the shelf and read it.

In the public sector, interoperability is a similarly crucial issue. This means that emergency plans between different levels in the same system (e.g. health organization at national, regional and local levels), between agencies (e.g. different government departments) and between neighbouring countries must ideally interlink and at least not conflict. Interoperability is very amenable to exploration and resolution through exercises.

6.4   Background to the Role of Exercises in Pandemic Preparedness

The UK has been very prominent internationally in using exercises to test and develop pandemic preparedness. It is therefore impossible to avoid such emphasis in this section; however, the underlying principles of exercises and exercise design are similar for all jurisdictions. Nevertheless, the way services in both the health sector and in related government departments operate and relate to each other may vary considerably from country to country. This section is not a detailed discussion of the operational aspects of running pandemic influenza exercises, but is intended to give the reader an understanding of how exercise methodologies can be used to develop and improve pandemic response.

For centuries military doctrine has stated that exercises (the use of simulated battle situations where troops and materiel are employed on manoeuvres) are a crucial part of the training and development of a military force. Philip of Macedon (reign 359–336 BC), father of Alexander the Great, was a keen advocate of this system, and his considerable military success is partially attributed to the thorough training of his armies. Military exercises can be used to test the operational aspects of a military unit but almost as importantly they can be used to test operational planning status and the command and control structure of a force.

Today the military and some other front-line responding services such as Fire and Rescue Services spend a considerable amount of time (over half in some services) exercising and training, and this has become an accepted and funded part of their work pattern. One of the main reasons for this is that through exercising activities repeatedly, staff can follow protocols and operate equipment in high-pressure, real-event situations in an efficient and effective manner. Exercises are an important part of the emergency planning cycle (Fig. 6.2), being an important tool to assess what has been learned from training and to identify components of a response that can rectified by amending plans or service configuration.

In the healthcare sector, the concept of specifically designing and running exercises to examine and explore responses to emergency situations either man-made (e.g. deliberate release of a toxic material) or natural (e.g. pandemic influenza) is relatively recent. In the UK most exercises prior to 2001 were small-scale and conducted within hospitals or ambulance services that have a statutory responsibility to exercise annually. In general, health services (apart from the Ambulance Service) were not routinely involved in large-scale multi-agency civil response exercises held up until the late 1990s.

After the events of 9/11 and the anthrax letters of autumn 2001 in the USA, there was a significant shift in thinking as it became apparent that a well-trained and

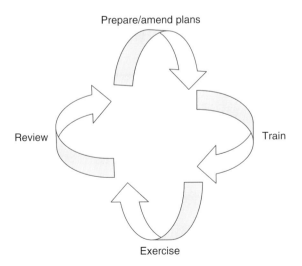

Fig. 6.2. The emergency planning cycle.

practised health service response would be crucial to optimizing the response to a deliberately released biological organism, noxious chemical or an explosive device containing the above. Therefore further funding was made available in the UK for the design and running of exercises to develop health responses to deliberate release incidents. The early exercises were successful, although some work had to be done to convince both clinicians and healthcare managers that these activities were a good use of staff time. When severe acute respiratory syndrome appeared in 2003, exercises were requested to assess how healthcare systems could respond to this threat. The success of exercises has made them an increasing part of the emergency preparedness and response culture in the UK healthcare system. Designing exercises to explore the operation of pandemic influenza plans began to happen in 2003, coinciding with an increase in the pace of pandemic preparedness activities, as influenza A/H5N1 re-emerged in South-east Asia. The underpinning rationale for performing exercises in a healthcare context is to:

- Create multi-agency links with relevant non-health organizations.
- Clarify roles and responsibilities between agencies and between tiers within organizations (e.g. primary and secondary care).
- Identify lessons and gaps in capability, which can then be rectified.
- Improve preparedness and response to health protection emergencies.
- Reinforce training and identify training gaps.

Although healthcare exercises are clearly a vital part of pandemic preparedness, it would be incorrect to paint an impression that these should occur in isolation of other sectors. Pandemic influenza is rightly regarded as a whole-of-society emergency that generates so many non-health issues (e.g. business continuity and maintenance of essential services) that it requires a coordinated, multi-sectoral approach (Chapter 11).

6.5 Types of Exercise

There are three main types of exercise design that can be used in a healthcare setting and examples of each with respect to pandemic influenza are discussed in this chapter. Rather like the three main types of epidemiological study, where each in turn is more appropriate for answering some types of questions than others, these three exercise designs are each best suited for testing different elements of pandemic response. They also vary in the resources needed to run them and the choice of exercise is important: it should provide the most appropriate and cost-effective way of achieving its aims and objectives.

One of the most important issues when organizing an exercise is to be very sure of the aims and objectives of the activity, i.e. what responses or functions are to be tested? This then allows the design of an appropriate and targeted exercise. A poorly designed and run exercise represents an expensive mistake which is often avoidable, and one of the commonest mistakes is not having clear aims and objectives.

Table-top exercises (desktop exercises)

'Table-top' or 'desktop' exercises (DTXs) are a very cost-effective and efficient method of testing plans, procedures and people; they are so named because they can literally be played sitting around a table or desk. Players from the participating agencies assemble in one place for a typical period of 1 or 2 days and play out in theory what would happen in practice, using specially designed scenarios. They are difficult to run with large numbers (150 is a sensible maximum), but those players who are involved are provided with an excellent opportunity to interact with, and understand, the roles and responsibilities of the other agencies taking part. A DTX can engage players imaginatively and generate high levels of realism. Participants will gain familiarity with key procedures along with the people with whom they may be working in an emergency, in a realistic fashion. Those who have exercised together and know each other will provide a much more effective response than those who come together for the first time when an incident occurs. An element of 'media play' (rehearsing, under pressure, what would be communicated to the media) can be introduced under controlled conditions, and this creates a lot of interest and realism, as well as pressure on participants!

The aims and objectives of many pandemic influenza exercises have been concerned not only with testing plans at various health service command and control levels, but also looking at how health plans integrate with partner agencies' plans, and consequently DTXs are often the most appropriate format of exercise to use. Depending on the complexity of the plans being tested and the number of agencies involved, some pandemic influenza DTXs have a complex structure of inter-agency relationships between organizational teams (called 'syndicates' in exercise terminology) and require careful planning and skilled facilitation. Where multiple agencies are involved, a multi-room venue is often best; this allows space for individual agencies to debate and formulate decisions in private, yet the proximity to other syndicates to facilitate 'exercise play'. An example is given in Fig. 6.3.

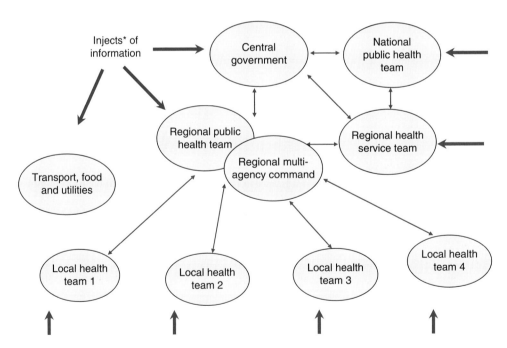

Fig. 6.3. Example of a desktop exercise (DTX) syndicate structure.
*An 'inject' is a piece of information deliberately given to some or all exercise participants (players) to stimulate activity or force decisions to be made.

J. Simpson and C. Sellwood

Because demand for pandemic influenza DTXs has rapidly outstripped the number of skilled exercise facilitators available, 'off-the-shelf' packages have now been produced. These packages have instructions on how to design and manage a simple DTX, sets of injects (questions to be answered or situations to be introduced during the course of the exercise) and DVD clips to introduce and move on the exercise play. These allow organizations to adopt a 'do-it-yourself' approach, and have proved very popular – in the UK one such package has been used by over 70 healthcare organizations. Some of these packages are available free from the WHO.

Command post exercises

In a command post exercise (denoted CPX), the organizations or teams (and communications teams) from each participating organization are positioned at the actual control posts or 'duty stations' they would use during a real incident. This tests communication arrangements and, more importantly, information flows between remotely positioned teams from participating organizations. A CPX is usually more realistic than a DTX because flaws in communications and information technology are readily exposed.

CPXs are especially good at examining how geographically distant organizations will communicate with each other; they are also very useful in testing data flows and the assembly of information for surveillance and reporting, although this requires considerable work in preparing 'dummy' data to test the systems. There have been a large number of international CPXs which have explored cross-jurisdiction communication especially in the early stages of a pandemic.

Field exercises (live exercises)

Field exercises involve deploying staff and assets in live play, and range from a small-scale test of one component of the response – like evacuation, ranging from a building or 'incident' site to an affected community – through to a full-scale test of the whole organization's response to an incident. Live exercises provide the best means of confirming the satisfactory operation of emergency communications, and the use of 'casualties' can add to the realism.

While large-scale field exercises to test the response to an avian influenza incident might be possible, testing a response to pandemic influenza in this way is not practical. However, field tests of individual components of the overall response have been undertaken in many countries. Examples of field exercise undertaken include looking at how hospital infection control procedures would work during an influenza pandemic, how a port health system would operate at an airport, and assessing the most efficient mode of operation of a mass prophylaxis centre distributing antiviral medication.

'Complex' exercises

Because of the severe societal issues raised by an influenza pandemic, many countries have held large, complex exercises to test their national influenza pandemic plan, using two or even all three of the above modalities to test the plan's operability on a nationwide basis (looking at the coordination of local, regional and national response). Such exercises are difficult and expensive to design and run, but are valuable in showing players including senior officials and government ministers how a pandemic might be managed and some of the complexities and nuances of the response needed. They are probably not the best starting option for governments and organizations that are new or inexperienced in conducting exercise. One such exercise held in 2007 in the UK, called Exercise Winter Willow, was the largest civil exercise in the UK since the end of the Cold War. With over 5000 participants from the local healthcare providers to the ministerial level, this exercise tested the command and control structures in the UK and helped identify areas for further planning. Exercise Cumpston 06 took place in Australia in 2006 to test pandemic response, and was the largest ever civil exercise undertaken in that country. Examples of major pandemic-specific issues that can be explored using exercises are:

- command, control and decision making by officials and ministers;
- health system response;
- use of public health countermeasures;
- ports and border issues;
- pharmaceutical countermeasures, including supply chain issues;
- vaccine availability and prioritization;
- simultaneous high-level sickness absence in all employment sectors;
- loss of key staff;
- food, fuel and power shortages/outages;
- infection control measures and use of protective equipment;
- civil disorder and panic;
- loss of mass transportation systems; and
- assistance to 'home' citizens stranded overseas.

Note that these are illustrative examples and not an exhaustive list.

6.6 Potential Problems in the Design of Pandemic Influenza Exercises

Interaction with expert advice

Pandemic influenza is a complex subject, and most people who are involved in exercise planning and design are generally more experienced in scenario writing and developing exercises that look at the response to other major acute events and not usually influenza experts. It is therefore of crucial importance to obtain advice and work closely with subject experts in the field to provide relevant and challenging scenarios for the exercises; likewise, experts in pandemic influenza must engage with exercise design teams to make the best of their specialist skills. For example, without an expert understanding of the medical science and policy aspects of human A/H5N1 vaccines, a generic exercise planner would have great difficulty in designing an exercise that tested critical decision making points regarding their potential deployment, and an exercise scenario based on a theoretical A/H7N3 pandemic virus would by definition rule out exercise play involving A/H5N1 vaccines. This example reinforces the need for careful definition of the aims and objectives.

J. Simpson and C. Sellwood

Time

An influenza pandemic is predicted to last about 4–5 months in any given country and, in general, exercises can be run in a healthcare setting for only 1 or 2 days due to staff availability. This (and the impossibility of providing meaningful exercise play lasting several months) means running an exercise exploring the whole pandemic response in real time is not an option. When exercises were first being designed to look at pandemic influenza response in the UK, there was a great emphasis on pre-pandemic to early pandemic activity. As there is now more confidence in the response to these phases, more recent exercises have progressed to focus on peak activity, with an emphasis on business continuity, or on the recovery phase. There has also been more emphasis on how certain parts of the system would respond in detail, for example exercises to test the pharmaceutical supply chain. Therefore various different designs have been developed so response across a pandemic wave can be explored.

The time block method

In this design the exercise is broken into three or more time blocks, each of which looks at issues that need to be addressed on a single day in the pandemic response. Often in a three-block design there have been blocks looking at: (i) the early stages of the pandemic; (ii) the peak of the pandemic; and (iii) the recovery phase. Each block usually lasts 2–3 h and it is important that before each block starts all players are certain where they are in respect to the pandemic timeline. This requires careful 'pre-loading' (i.e. building up the scenario or the story) using written materials and recorded DVDs, for example, using simulated news broadcasts to 'set' players' minds to the correct time. Most DTXs looking at pandemic influenza response use this methodology.

Running half-day or 1 day per week over multiple weeks

In this methodology each session explores a half-day or whole day in the pandemic response each week for, say, 8–12 weeks. This gives a very good sense of the protracted length of the response needed with respect to pandemic influenza and is achievable in a command post format. It does, however, require considerable resources to design and run, also considerable commitment from participating organizations because of the need to release staff from their normal duties to play the exercise for up to 1 day per week, for up to 12 consecutive weeks.

Run the exercise for 2 to 4 days in real time, playing out part of 1 week of the response

This again is suitable for command post format and was the methodology for Exercise Winter Willow mentioned above. It does give some idea of the intensity, complexity and need for sustainability in the response to an influenza pandemic and is more easily achievable than the second methodology. However, it is probably not the best format for governments and organizations that are new or inexperienced in conducting exercises.

Scene setting

Pandemic influenza exercises need data on attack rates, morbidity and mortality rates, sickness absence and hospitalization, etc. in order to make the exercise scenarios plausible and challenging. Many pandemic influenza exercises are therefore built around a mathematical model that can provide these data. In the UK the model often used is a simplified model with a single pandemic wave which gives a good approximation of real data but is easy and quick to run (most planning models are difficult to use and take a significant time to produce data).

6.7 Lessons Identified

One of the major reasons for running an exercise is to identify gaps in plans and capabilities, which can then be reported to the relevant organizations and authorities for remedies to be devised, thus allowing completion of the emergency planning cycle (Fig. 6.2). It is important that any exercise is evaluated fully and a report written and disseminated; there are many detailed methodologies for analysing the outcome of exercises, but these lie outside the scope of this book. It is important that the lessons are reported against the aims and objectives, as the aims in a large command post national exercise will be very different from those of a small field exercise looking at infection control on a ward. This is one of the reasons why the setting accurate, realistic and achievable aims and objectives is so important in exercise design. It is also important to have follow-up activity after exercises (6 months later) to ascertain whether lessons identified have been followed up by changes in policy and procedure. Some generic lessons identified from pandemic influenza exercises performed by the Health Protection Agency in the UK and abroad in 2007, of interest to an international audience, are:

- Increased communication between health and non-health agencies at all levels is essential. At present in many countries the only formal communication between the sectors is at national level. Regular contact between both sectors at local, regional, national and international levels will facilitate better working in an emergency.
- The cooperation within and between local, regional and national organizations should be developed and improved. There should be a clear chain of command and communication from top down (national to local level) and bottom up (local to national level).
- Further consideration is needed on the burial of the dead and school closures during a pandemic, which have both emerged repeatedly as problem areas.
- The rapid development and production of a pandemic strain vaccine and its dissemination is key, as is the need for international cooperation over this issue.
- There is a lack of detailed guidance available on the recovery phase of a pandemic. Over the last few years, much work has been done regionally, nationally and

J. Simpson and C. Sellwood

internationally on pandemic preparedness, which has involved health and multi-agency planning and exercising at all levels. However, plans in place focus primarily on the preparedness and response phases of a pandemic without much consideration of how 'a return to normality' might be achieved.

- Many organizations are unclear about their priorities at the end of a pandemic. This is not surprising as it is difficult to predict what position they will be in or what resources will be available. The impact on business continuity, particularly of the health service, is likely to be prolonged and severe. However, the demand for services to return to normal as quickly as possible following a pandemic is likely to be considerable.

6.8 Conclusion

Influenza pandemics pose one of the greatest infectious disease threats to mankind. It is possible to learn from previous pandemics, other infectious disease outbreaks and other civil emergencies to be able to plan for such an event. Planning needs to be undertaken at all levels, from international down to individual organizations and companies. Formal BCP is an essential element of this process. If not addressed, unforeseen interdependencies and lack of interoperability within and between organizations present a major potential vulnerability.

Planning for the response to pandemic influenza has been important in the evolution of civil exercises. Such exercises are now considered an integral and acceptable element of pandemic preparedness in many countries. Novel methodologies have been developed to cope with the particular scientific challenges of the pandemic response.

6.9 Summary Points

- Pandemic preparedness addresses a 'rising tide' event that lasts over an extended period of time with little scope for mutual aid, whereas more standard emergency preparedness plans are aimed at 'big bang' events where the duration of the incident is likely to be short-lived (although the full response may take longer) and mutual aid is more likely to be available.
- An influenza pandemic will affect all sectors of society over an extended period of time. The impact of such an extended interruption should be considered through generic BCP in the first instance. Issues which cannot be addressed through BCP should then be considered individually.
- Pandemic influenza generates many non-health issues (e.g. business continuity issues due to high levels of staff absence). The whole-of-society effect means exercises are much more valuable when they explore a coordinated, multi-agency approach.
- The extended length of time of an influenza pandemic wave means real-time exercising is appropriate only for exploring issues over a small part of the pandemic event. To address this, methodologies have been developed to allow coherent play across the time span of a pandemic wave such as the time block methodology.
- There has been a great demand for exercises to explore pandemic influenza responses. The limited number of expert staff available cannot design and run exercises for every organization that wishes to run one, and have needed to

concentrate on designing the more complex exercises with a wide scope. An 'off-the-shelf' package, designed by a specialist unit, allows organizations to run a more simple exercise design using their own staff resources and expertise.

Further Reading

Australian Government, Department of Health and Ageing, Office of Health Protection (2007) *National Pandemic Influenza Exercise. Operation Cumpston 06 Report.* http://www.health.gov.au/internet/panflu/publishing.nsf/Content/34B24A2E2E6018E9CA2573D700 0006D2/$File/exercise-cumpston-report.pdf (accessed May 2009).

British Standards Institution (2006) BS 25999-1:2006. *Business continuity management – Part 1, Code of Practice.* http://www.bsi-global.com/en/Assessment-and-certification-services/management-systems/Standards-and-Schemes/BS-25999/ (accessed May 2009).

European Commission and UK Health Protection Agency (2006) *A pandemic exercise for the European Union.* Exercise Common Ground, Serial 5.0, Final Report. http://ec.europa.eu/health/ph_threats/com/common.pdf (accessed May 2009).

HM Government (2009) *How prepared are you? Business Continuity Management Toolkit, Version 1.* http://www.direct.gov.uk/en/Governmentcitizensandrights/Dealingwithemergencies/Preparingforemergencies/DG_175927 (accessed May 2009).

Phin, N.F., Rylands, A.J., Allan, J., Edwards, C., Enstone, J.E. and Nguyen-Van-Tam, J.S. (2009) Personal protective equipment in an influenza pandemic: a UK simulation exercise. *Journal of Hospital Infection* 71, 15–21.

UK Cabinet Office (2006) *Contingency planning for a possible influenza pandemic, Version 2.* http://www.cabinetoffice.gov.uk/media/132467/060710_revised_pandemic.pdf (accessed May 2009)

UK Cabinet Office (2009) *Exercise Winter Willow and other UK pandemic influenza exercises.* http://www.cabinetoffice.gov.uk/ukresilience/pandemicflu/exercises.aspx (accessed May 2009).

United Nations Office for the Coordination of Humanitarian Affairs (2007) *Pandemic Influenza Contingency. 39 Steps Governments Should Take to Prepare for a Pandemic.* http://www.un-pic.org/pic/web/documents/english/39%20Steps%20Governments%20Should%20Take%20To%20Prepare%20for%20Pandemic.pdf (accessed May 2009).

World Health Organization (2005) *WHO Global Influenza Preparedness Plan. The role of WHO and recommendations for national measures before and during pandemics.* http://www.who.int/csr/resources/publications/influenza/WHO_CDS_CSR_GIP_2005_5.pdf (accessed May 2009).

7 Bio-mathematical Modelling (What Will and Won't Work)

P.G. GROVE

- What is modelling and what is its role in pandemic preparedness?
- What can modelling tell us and what can't it tell us?
- How does the discipline work?
- What is real-time prediction?
- How much confidence should we have in modelling?

7.1 What is Modelling?

The word 'modelling' is used to describe many diverse activities even within the scientific disciplines. However, the essence is to use one's broad knowledge of whatever system is under consideration to construct a simplified or idealized version, the 'model'. The model can then be analysed in detail, frequently, and in practice most usefully, using often complex mathematical techniques.

Why build a model? There are basically two reasons. The first is that broad knowledge of a given system is not sufficient to describe the detail that needs to be considered. The second is that even if every detail were known, the very amount of information would make it hard to handle and impractical to work out what was going on. Of course it is necessary to include 'significant detail', and the choice of what is 'significant' in this respect depends on our broad knowledge of the system in question and on judgement. Modelling is thus not an alternative to having knowledge about a system; rather it is a way of sorting knowledge to determine the relative importance of various factors and re-ordering the information to provide answers which are not always immediately obvious. For example, grossly oversimplifying, infectious disease modelling involves attempting to predict the total number of people who will be infected by a disease from the number of people one person infects and how quickly that infection takes place.

As the 'significant' detail will, in general, depend on the question being asked, different questions will require different simplifications. Hence many different models are usually required to capture the different aspects of a complicated problem. Thus knowledge of how a particular model fails to capture all the aspects of the real situation is at least as important as the model itself.

A large component of the 'broad knowledge' required for biomedical modelling is, of course, the germ theory of disease, in particular, medical knowledge of how the disease is passed from one person to another, along with our knowledge of the effects on that person and the results of treatment of various kinds. Of course, in relation to influenza, many of the details of how the infection is transmitted are poorly understood (Chapter 5), posing additional challenges. The other important component is information on how people interact: how often do they meet and how often do they travel from place to place?

A corollary of all this is that modelling can only be as good as the data fed into the models and the assumptions made in the design of the models. As earlier chapters have indicated, in the case of dealing with a future pandemic influenza virus, there are few specific data and a wide range of plausible assumptions. Therefore, the role of modelling prior to a pandemic cannot be to make definitive forecasts of what will happen. If this is the case, why is modelling essential to planning for a pandemic?

What modelling can do is: (i) help map out the range of possible risks; and, more importantly, (ii) suggest which responses are robust over the range of uncertainty.

Put another way, modelling can help determine how bad a pandemic might be and see which interventions have a reasonable chance of improving the situation. Indeed, it is essentially the only way of seeing which interventions (or combinations of interventions) will have any chance of working across the range of uncertainty.

7.2   How Bad Might a Pandemic Be?

Modelling helps map out the range of possible risks by providing a description of how quickly a pandemic would move across the world and what would happen if a pandemic arrived in, say, the UK, assuming no interventions. The modelling is based on empirical information from past pandemics and seasonal influenza of the kind described in earlier chapters. The objective of this kind of analysis is to indicate the scale of the problems involved in dealing with a pandemic.

It would be wrong to think that the assessment of how severe a pandemic might be comes solely from modelling. The real value of modelling in this aspect of planning is to cross-check and to integrate various different sources of information. For example, the rate of increase of the number of clinical cases of influenza in the second wave of the 1918 pandemic in both the UK and the USA suggests that one person infected about two others (a figure called R_0). Modelling then tells us that in a fully susceptible population, 80% of the population might become infected (the infection attack rate). Information from seasonal influenza suggests that between 50 and 66% of the cases might show significant clinical symptoms, which combined with the 80% infection attack rate gives a resultant clinical attack rate of up to 50%. On the other hand, information from previous pandemics suggests clinical attack rates in the general community of up to 40%. Thus the various ways of looking at past data suggest that it would be reasonable to plan for 'reasonable worst case' clinical attack rates in the range of 40 to 50%.

One can also use empirical information from past pandemics and seasonal influenza to estimate the case fatality and hospitalization rates. This is often difficult owing to the way the data were originally collected. Another use of modelling is to construct a model of the community from which the data came in order to help understand if the way the data were collected may have either inflated or deflated the estimates. Once estimates of case fatality and hospitalization are obtained, these can be combined with the clinical attack rate to see if services would be overcome by the demand.

The next step is to look at the disease spread. There are three aspects:

- How quickly would it arrive in Europe or the UK (assuming its origin, say, in South-east Asia)?
- How quickly would it spread though a given land mass, for example the UK or mainland Europe?
- What would be the timing of the epidemic both nationally and locally?

Again, empirical data exist from previous pandemics (seasonal flu data are less useful because of the low susceptibility of the population); however, transport and communications, especially international transport, have changed greatly even since the 1968 pandemic and do not in themselves provide a good guide. The models can accommodate these changes in travel patterns and indicate what would have happened in 1918 or 1957 had there been modern-day patterns of travel.

We have stressed that modelling does not replace knowledge but rather allows it to be used more efficiently. Modelling the worldwide spread of a pandemic can be done, but a fundamental lack of understanding means that there is an important aspect of a pandemic for which modelling cannot provide answers. This is the question of pandemic 'waves' (Chapter 4). Modellers can generate pandemics with waves, for example by assuming a seasonal effect on the transmission of influenza; however, none of the suggested mechanisms can explain all the observations. Without this basic understanding, modelling cannot provide us with further insight. Fortunately, for most planning purposes a single wave is the 'worst case' with the greatest number of people becoming sick or requiring hospitalization at any one time.

7.3 What Might Work?

The second role of modelling is to help find 'robust' packages of interventions. There are two stages to this. The first is to separate those interventions that are expected to have some useful impact across the range of uncertainty from those that would have an insignificant impact and/or an impact only in very specific circumstances. Only modelling can do this. One reason for this is that many of the most important interventions such as antiviral drugs and vaccines have not been available in previous pandemics. Also, the context of interventions such as travel restrictions has changed significantly since the last pandemic. Modelling is also needed to disentangle the effects of interventions used in combination in the past and use this information to assess the different combinations one would wish to use in a future pandemic. Equally important is the fact that only modelling allows consideration of the effects of the interventions for pandemics of different severity.

Some interventions can be shown to be essentially worthless at any practical level of implementation – in particular travel restrictions. Others can be shown to be more effective than one might imagine, for example, a poorly matched pre-pandemic vaccine which reduced transmission (by reducing the probability of being infected) by only 20% would have a significant impact on a pandemic.

A close relative of epidemiological modelling is 'operational' modelling. This kind of modelling investigates if there are practical ways of implementing the countermeasures that are shown to be effective in conventional epidemiological studies. Only if some practical route of implementation exists (i.e. the intervention can be properly delivered at the 'coal face') can a countermeasure be considered to 'work'.

Some interventions, such as some kinds of social distancing measures, tend to be effective only at low values of R_0 and hence they do not in themselves turn out to be robust measures. Some such as school closures do not have a great deal of impact in themselves, but seem to offer important adjunct effects when used alongside other measures such as household prophylaxis (Chapters 8 and 10).

This indicates one particularly important feature of modelling: it allows us to consider several measures in combination. We can therefore consider packages of measures in which we can not only consider the situation where they all work as expected, but also where some measures fail. Reasons for possible failure include:

- Antiviral prophylaxis failing to have the anticipated effect because drugs do not get to people quickly enough.
- Antiviral treatment failing due to the emergence of drug resistance.
- Antibiotic treatment failing because most complications are not bacterial.

Packages can therefore be designed to be robust not only because each individual measure has a reasonable possibility of working across the range of uncertainty, but also because if one measure fails the other parts of the package should still have a significant impact on the epidemic of pandemic influenza.

However, it should be strongly re-emphasized that these calculations do not constitute forecasts of what will happen. Rather they indicate the kinds of effects the different measures might be expected to produce and hence the ways in which they are best included in the package. The point of the exercise is to come up with combinations that will probably work despite the fact that we cannot accurately estimate the effect of each element.

7.4 What Do the Models Look Like?

The simplest epidemiological model that reproduces the most important qualitative features of epidemics is the deterministic homogeneous mixing SIA or SIR model (Fig. 7.1).

The population is broken down into three groups: those susceptible (S) who have not been infected or are not yet infectious; an infectious group (I); and an attacked (A) group who have either recovered (R) or died. As it is most likely to be the case with pandemic influenza that most people recover, this is often called an SIR model (as shown in Fig. 7.1). Members of the susceptible population have an equal chance of being infected by a member of the infectious population and in turn becoming infectious. The average flows between the groups are described by 'non-linear differential' equations, which essentially means that people are treated as a kind of 'fluid' that moves between the groups and the calculations are analogous to the 'bath-

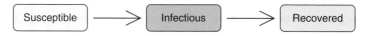

Fig. 7.1. SIR model (the SIA model where all recover).

filling problems' of secondary school calculus courses. The mathematically inclined reader may have been alerted to the 'non-linear' description of the differential equations; the implications of this will be discussed later.

Given its simplicity, the basic SIA model gives a remarkable degree of insight into how epidemics behave, but it is easily extendable to give more realistic representations. The S, I and A groups can be broken down by, say, age or geographical region, and members of each group then meet and/or infect people of different ages and regions at different rates. Additional groups can also be introduced, such as those infected or ill but not (so) infectious. It is possible to get away from treating people as a fluid, but instead as individuals introducing a probability of infection – creating a so-called 'stochastic model'. Such stochastic models are particularly important in considering the early evolution of an epidemic. One common approach to infectious disease modelling is to build up from an SIA model of the kind described to a level of complexity that captures the problem at hand.

An alternative approach is to start not at the level of a population group but of the individual, an approach pioneered in the UK by Ferguson and colleagues at Imperial College London. Here a model is constructed of each person who travels from home to work or school, or across or out of the country by delivering goods or going on holiday. Because of the limitations of data the individuals are (at least conceptually) bunched into groups with similar behaviour. Additional complexity is introduced into this model by adding more groups with a wider range of different behaviours.

Which approach is better? The simple answer is that we need both approaches. The individual-level approach is much more flexible than the SIA-based approach. It is much easier to test out strategies such as the post-exposure prophylaxis of households or the isolation and/or quarantine of cases in a model that considers individuals. On the other hand, the sheer complexity of an individual-based model makes it difficult to see the implications of the large number of assumptions that have had to be made in the construction of the model. In an SIA approach the implications of the few necessary assumptions are clear.

The need to understand the impact of the assumptions of the model is particularly important because of the 'non-linear' nature of the models mentioned earlier. This has two implications. The first is that it is impossible to write down an explicit formula for, say, the number of people who will get ill on any given day, even for the very simplest SIA model. A computer can approximate the curve for a specific case but this is very different to knowing what will happen in general (particularly important when dealing with a new virus). The second is that small changes in the parameters (i.e. the numbers which describe the model like R_0) do not just produce small quantitative changes in the results, but can change the entire qualitative behaviour of the model. Such changes can be tested for, and explored, by investigating the effects of changing the parameters (so-called 'sensitivity analysis'). More seriously, small differences in assumptions of the structure of the model can have similarly large qualitative effects and there is no systematic method analogous to 'sensitivity analysis' to test for such effects.

This critical dependence on assumptions impacts on the two families of models in different ways. In the SIA type of approach the 'significant detail' may not be obvious and small effects that have a significant effect on the results may have been ignored. Fortunately, SIA models seem to be relatively robust against small changes in parameter and/or assumption. On the other hand, in the individual approach there are so many implicit assumptions that there is a considerable chance of implicitly making one which changes the results significantly. The structural stability of such models in the epidemiological sphere is currently poorly understood.

These considerations mean that it is, at least initially, essential to compare the results of many models to draw any conclusions from epidemiological modelling. Only after obtaining a consensus that a particular approach, or set of approaches, is appropriate is it possible to construct a model that can be used to produce results similar to the consensus view over a limited range. Even then, some divergence in views is possible if there is no agreement on the parameters of the model. This is especially the case if parameters have been derived by seeing which parameters allow models to describe historical epidemics. On the other hand, different models may suggest very different parameters for historical epidemics but agree on the impact of countermeasures in a future pandemic because the difference in parameters compensates for the different assumptions in building the models.

From a policy maker's perspective, if SIA and 'individual' modelling approaches offer the same general conclusions, this increases confidence about making the correct decision in critical areas, although it does not guarantee the eventual outcome. Thus pandemic policy making needs to be based on the expert consensus of results from of a number of different models. In the UK a 'modelling' group reporting to the Cabinet Office has been set up for this purpose.

7.5 Economic Models

This chapter has been concerned mainly with epidemiological modelling. We have mentioned briefly the operational modelling required to see if countermeasures are practical in the sense that if, for example, the epidemiological modelling assumes everyone who is ill will be treated with antivirals, it is via some means possible to treat everyone. Another measure of practicality is economic impact. Outputs of the epidemiological modelling are the numbers of deaths, hospitalizations and cases both with and without intervention. These can be placed in standard economics frameworks to assess the cost–benefit of packages on intervention.

Health interventions are usually measured by the cost-effectiveness ratio of the cost to gain a quality-adjusted life year (QALY). If the cost is much in excess of £30,000 per QALY an intervention is highly likely to be rejected. However, the impact of a pandemic is more than simply the health impact measured in QALYs. Instead, attempts are made to produce money estimates of health impacts which can be added to, say, estimates of production lost due to those at home ill or looking after sick children. Precisely what can be estimated and/or should be included differ from one analysis to another, but it is clear that if the annual probability of a pandemic is in the range of 1 to 3% then the standard UK cross-government estimates for the money value of death, hospitalization and lost output would make the use of antivirals, pre-pandemic vaccine and antibiotics strongly cost beneficial.

7.6 Real-time Modelling

This chapter has so far emphasized that, before a future pandemic arrives, one cannot attempt forecasting because there is simply too wide a range of possibilities as to how the pandemic will evolve. As information becomes available in a pandemic, however,

P.G. Grove

Focus Box 7.1. A selection of the most influential papers modelling pandemic influenza.

Containment

- Ferguson, N.M., Cummings, D.A., Cauchemez, S., Fraser, C., Riley, S., Meeyai, A., Iamsirithaworn, S. and Burke, D.S. (2005) Strategies for containing an emerging influenza pandemic in Southeast Asia. *Nature* 437, 209–214.
- Longini, I.M., Halloran, M.E., Nizam, A. and Yang, Y. (2004) Containing pandemic influenza with antiviral agents. *American Journal of Epidemiology* 159, 623–633.

Using individual based models, these papers indicate that, if the first incipient pandemic cases are in a rural part of South-east Asia, stringent social distance measures, the use of area quarantine and the implementation of a geographically based, large-scale, antiviral prophylaxis policy could contain an outbreak with up to three million courses of antivirals for R_0 of up to about 2. Even if the strategy fails to contain the disease, it might delay its progress by about a month.

Entry screening

- Pitman, R.J., Cooper, B.S., Trotter, C.L., Gay, N.J. and Edmunds, W.J. (2005) Entry screening for severe acute respiratory syndrome (SARS) or influenza: policy evaluation. *British Medical Journal* 331, 1242–1243.

This paper considers the value of entry screening, given that passengers have been screened before starting their journey. The authors show that entry screening is unlikely to be effective in preventing the importation of either SARS or influenza. In the case of influenza the rapid rise in the number infected by those missed by the screening rapidly compensates for those identified by the screening. Combined with the results of Cooper *et al.* (2006), see below, this paper shows that no form of screening, entry or exit, will have a significant impact on the international spread of the pandemic.

International spread

- Cooper, B.S., Pitman, R.J., Edmunds, W.J. and Gay, N.J. (2006) Delaying the international spread of pandemic influenza. *PLoS Medicine* 3, 212.

Cooper and co-workers show that having taken 2–4 weeks to build up in the country of origin, pandemic flu could take as little as 2–4 weeks to spread from Asia to the UK, with the peak of the UK epidemic following about 50 days later. Imposing a 90% restriction on all air travel to the UK would delay the peak of a pandemic wave by only 1–2 weeks. On the other hand, a 99.9% travel restriction might delay a pandemic wave by 2 months but is probably impractical. The model is based on a SIA model of each major city, with infectious people being moved between cities according to the airline timetables.

Mitigation

- Ferguson, N.M., Cummings, D.A., Fraser, C., Cajka, J.C., Cooley, P.C. and Burke, D.S. (2006) Measures for mitigating an influenza pandemic. *Nature* 442, 448–452.

continued

Focus Box 7.1. **Continued.**

This paper is a portmanteau of numerous results for an epidemic from the Imperial College individual-based model. The results have been generally confirmed by other approaches but the Ferguson *et al.* (2006) paper remains a good summary. The most important results are as follows. Uncontained, a flu outbreak would be expected to spread to all major UK centres of population within 1–2 weeks. Because of probable multiple importations of pandemic influenza and the concentration of the population in cities, attempts at containment by targeted antiviral prophylaxis and practical social distance measures are very unlikely to succeed. Mass treatment of clinical cases with antivirals would flatten the temporal profile, lowering the peak and lengthening the base. Although the main purpose of antiviral treatment is to reduce the severity of the disease, treating all clinical cases with antivirals might also decrease the overall attack rate. To obtain a substantial effect the drug must be administered within 24 h of the start of symptoms. Post-exposure antiviral prophylaxis of the household contacts of cases could have a more marked impact on the disease than simply treatment of cases. Prior vaccination with a poorly matched (pre-pandemic) vaccine and antibiotic treatment of those with complications would also be important in controlling the overall impact on hospitalizations and deaths.

School closures

- Cauchemez, S., Valleron, A.J., Boëlle, P.Y., Flahault, A. and Ferguson, N.M. (2008) Estimating the impact of school closure on influenza transmission from sentinel data. *Nature* 452, 750–755.

The impact of closing schools, especially without any antiviral intervention, depends critically on the mixing between children and adults. Different plausible models give different results. This paper, based on the evidence from the closure of French schools during seasonal flu, suggests a maximum possible reduction in the peak incidence of one half and rather less in practice. In any case the reduction in the total number of cases is rather less, at most 20%.

UK Scientific Pandemic Influenza Committee Modelling Sub-Group – modelling summary

Government preparations for a pandemic cannot wait for the publication of results in the academic literature. A great deal of unpublished modelling has been considered by the UK Scientific Pandemic Influenza Committee Modelling Sub-Group. A summary of these results is available online (http://www.dh.gov.uk/ab/SPI/index.htm).

forecasting will begin to become possible. Indeed short-term forecasting will even be necessary to make sense of what is happening 'now', a process known as 'nowcasting'. This is because data on influenza-like illness (ILI) will initially be swamped by the usual background of ILI rather than genuine pandemic cases. In addition, there are the natural delays between illness and eventual death that make fatality rates difficult to calculate, as well as straightforward reporting delays of various kinds. These effects will need to be removed in the process of making short-term forecasts. These forecasts will therefore provide the best estimate of what is happening 'now' as well as over the next few days.

P.G. Grove

That such forecasting and nowcasting should become possible as the pandemic progresses is fortunate, because for some of the (otherwise robust) interventions, there are aspects of their use which can only be decided on the basis of the actual behaviour of the particular pandemic. Examples are the selection of antiviral policy (i.e. treatment or prophylaxis) given a limited antiviral stockpile and whether or not schools should be closed to reduce transmission. To manage these aspects of the response to an epidemic effectively it will be necessary to both understand what is happening at the time (in terms of cases deaths, hospitalizations, etc.) and be able to predict the total numbers expected over the course of the epidemic. This knowledge will need to be based on 'within-pandemic' or 'real-time' modelling using timely and accurate surveillance data.

In the particular case of antivirals policy, the largest impact is gained by, in the first instance, the most widespread distribution policy possible with the antiviral stockpile available (e.g. household prophylaxis for stockpiles greater than 50% of the population or universal treatment for stockpiles less than 50%) and then reverting to more restrictive policies if supplies become limited. The decision to restrict use will need to be taken on the basis of the nowcasts and forecasts available at critical points in the pandemic showing how many antiviral courses will be required and to whom they are most usefully targeted.

Similarly, closing schools may produce large levels of absenteeism as parents need to stay at home to look after their children. Estimates made by the UK government (based on the country's social and occupational structure) suggest that peak work-force absenteeism could be doubled if schools are closed and that this policy is best used either to support antiviral prophylaxis (which would compensate for the additional absenteeism by reducing absenteeism due to illness) or with antiviral treatment if children are particularly badly affected. The actual effects on children can hence only be determined in the pandemic as a result of nowcasts.

Thus, to support both decisions, real-time modelling producing both: (i) 'nowcasts' (reflecting the best estimate of the current situation); and (ii) long-term forecasts of the epidemic will be required.

As has been described, 'nowcasts' will provide the best picture of the progress of the epidemic and provide information on the details of, say, who is most badly affected and hence the best targeting of antiviral treatment and whether schools should be closed. On the other hand, the essential information to inform policy decisions on antiviral policy (e.g. if targeting will be required) within an epidemic will come from long-term forecasts of cases and antiviral usage. The importance of having accurate forecasts is indicated by the fact that making the 'wrong' choice on antiviral policy might lead to a 50% increase in the number of deaths.

In the early stages of the pandemic in the UK there will still be very few data to use in real-time modelling. This will include some data from abroad along with epidemiological and serological information from contact tracing of the first few hundred UK cases. As the epidemic continues, aggregate data, principally from the telephone-based antiviral assessment system, will begin to emerge. It will, however, be a challenge to extract the essential parameters even from the aggregate data until relatively late.

For some time into the pandemic, therefore, the long-term forecasts will predict a considerable range of outcomes and decision making will need to be made in 'windows' when the available information becomes just sufficient to inform the necessary decisions at that stage of the epidemic. In real-time modelling, just as in pre-pandemic modelling, it will be important to have alternative models and to compare and discuss the results.

7.7 How Much Confidence Should We Have in Modelling?

There are two basic errors in considering modelling results. One is to believe them, the other is not to believe them. Even in the most complicated non-linear system, good data and lots of trial and error will eventually produce a model that is predictive most of the time. A good example of this is weather forecasting, where decades of effort and a new trial every day have led to remarkably good short-term forecasting. A vast amount of time and effort, however, has been required to get weather forecasting to this condition, and even now forecast accuracy deteriorates rapidly over a short period of days into the future.

On the other hand, simple models that do not take account of the true complexity of a non-linear system are likely to be totally misleading and even more dangerous in public health terms. Models are most believable if they have resulted from a process in which different models have been compared and improved on the basis of the comparison – and if they are based on a sufficiently good set of data. To determine a 'good' model, one thus needs to be able to talk to the modeller who developed it. In this respect, simple Internet-based 'modelling toolkits' are fraught with problems (even if derived from reputable sources) and can give only the most superficial indication of what might happen.

As we have seen, there are currently few data to put into pandemic models and one should believe only those results that are couched in very general terms – 'this might do some good', 'this will not'. It is an equally safe assumption that any detailed predictions will prove to be wrong. However, if the models have been put together carefully, and their results compared systematically, then these general predictions are likely to be a good guide to what will happen. Good 'within-pandemic' or 'real-time' modelling will be based on models that not only make predictions but also estimate the uncertainty of their predictions, again by the comparison with the results of different models. If the models agree, and their estimated uncertainties fall as real data become available, they can be expected to give a reasonable forecast of what will happen.

In summary, modelling is an essential tool in preparing for, and understanding what will happen in, a pandemic. Without modelling results it would be impossible to judge which policies would be likely to be beneficial in a pandemic. Real-time modelling will also be essential in a pandemic but reliant on the input of high-quality epidemiological data as the pandemic unfolds. On the other hand, good modellers will be careful to explain that in the case of a pandemic their results are limited because of the lack of data and the limited scope for testing assumptions. Good pandemic planning is possible when the modellers are integral to the planning process and can explain what can and cannot be safely concluded from the modelling results.

7.8 Conclusion

Because we have limited experience of pandemics, and because we cannot predict with accuracy the behaviour of a future pandemic influenza virus, our preparations must depend on modelling results. These results can tell us which preparations are likely to work and which are likely to be of little value. On the other hand, modelling cannot make detailed forecasts of what will happen and plans need to be flexible to take account of this uncertainty.

7.9   Summary Points

- Mathematical epidemiological 'modelling' is the construction of a simplified description of the transmission of disease in a population, which can be analysed mathematically.
- Modelling can only be as good as the assumptions made in constructing the model and the parameters used in the numerical description. For a pandemic virus there are few data and a large range of plausible assumptions. We cannot, therefore, make forecasts of what will happen in a pandemic. The role of modelling before a pandemic is to tell us how bad a pandemic might be, and what countermeasures have a realistic possibility of having a significant effect across the large range of uncertainty about the nature and behaviours of the pandemic virus.
- Modelling is not about simply building a model and then 'running it' to find the answer. Reliable results need to be based on a consensus of the views of different modellers using different models. Off-the-shelf (or 'off-the-Internet') models should be treated with caution.
- When real data about the virus and its spread begin to appear in a pandemic, then forecasting of the progress of the pandemic becomes possible. Such forecasts (and the short-term versions known as 'nowcasts') have an important role in managing pandemic response.
- Models are not 'oracles' that can give definite predictions of the future, but properly used have an important role in helping to prepare for, and possibly managing the response to, a pandemic.

Further Reading

Anderson, R.M. and May, R.M. (1991) *Infectious Diseases of Humans.* Oxford University Press, Oxford, UK.

Daley, D.J. and Gani, J. (1999) *Epidemic Modelling.* Cambridge University Press, Cambridge, UK.

UK Cabinet Office, Civil Contingencies Secretariat (2007) *Overarching Government Strategy to respond to Pandemic Influenza – Analysis of the scientific evidence base.* http://www.cabinetoffice.gov.uk/media/131651/flu_pandemic_science_paper1.pdf (accessed May 2009).

UK Scientific Pandemic Influenza Committee (SPI) Subgroup on Modelling (2008) *Modelling Summary.* http://www.advisorybodies.doh.gov.uk/spi/minutes/spi-m-modellingsummary.pdf (accessed May 2009).

Pharmaceutical Interventions

J. VAN-TAM AND R.K. GUPTA

- What antiviral drugs are available to treat influenza?
- What will be their most likely public health benefits during a pandemic?
- Which antiviral drugs should be stockpiled?
- Is there a role for antibiotics in pandemic preparedness?
- Which antibiotics should be stockpiled?

8.1   Introduction

Since a pandemic-specific vaccine will not be available for several months after a pandemic has begun (Chapter 9), attention has focused on whether it is feasible to offer large-scale treatment against influenza. This includes treatment of the primary virus infection and subsequent bacterial complications if these occur. This chapter discusses currently available influenza antiviral drugs, relevant antibiotics, and their potential for stockpiling and use in a pandemic.

8.2   Antiviral Drugs

Several antiviral drugs are licensed for the treatment of influenza (Table 8.1). All of these drugs work by blocking a step in the replication cycle of the influenza virus, either at the point where the virus inserts its RNA into the host cell nucleus (M2-channel blockers) or at the point where newly formed viruses are released from the infected host cell (neuraminidase inhibitors) (Fig. 8.1). Detailed information on the influenza replication cycle is available in Chapter 2.

Two other antiviral drugs are of relevance. Ribavirin (Virazole®) is a broad-spectrum antiviral agent licensed for the treatment of respiratory syncytial virus by aerosol or nebulizer; however, it is also active against influenza and in controlled studies reduced the duration of fever and symptoms by about 1 day compared with placebo. Peramivir is a second-generation neuraminidase inhibitor which is currently still under development; although clinical development of an oral formulation has been halted, it will most likely be available for intravenous or intramuscular administration. Both of these drugs will be difficult to deploy outside hospitals and therefore have limited scope for mass deployment during a pandemic, but they might still have role in severely ill patients, especially peramivir. Finally, Symmetrel® is another brand of amantadine, but is currently licensed only for the treatment of Parkinson's disease.

©CAB International 2010. *Introduction to Pandemic Influenza*
(eds J.S. Nguyen-Van-Tam and C. Sellwood)

Table 8.1. Drugs licensed for the treatment of influenza.

Class	M2-channel blockers (adamantane)		Neuraminidase inhibitors	
Agent	Amantadine	Rimantadine	Zanamivir	Oseltamivir
Trade name	Lysovir®, Symadine®	Flumadine®	Relenza®	Tamiflu®
Influenza activity	A viruses only	A viruses only	A and B viruses	A and B viruses
Route of administration	Oral	Oral	Oral inhalation	Oral
Use for treatment	Yes	Yes	Yes	Yes
Use for prophylaxis	Yes	Yes	Yes	Yes

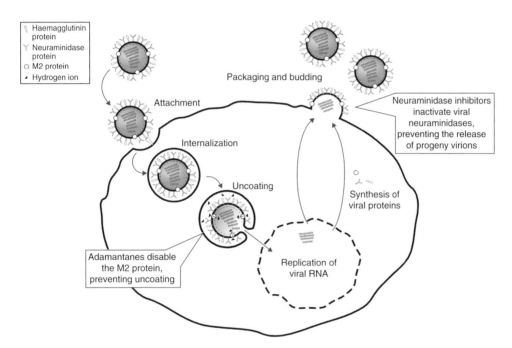

Fig. 8.1. Diagram showing points of action of M2-channel blockers and neuraminidase inhibitors in the replication cycle of influenza virus. (Kindly supplied by F. Hoffman-La Roche Ltd, Basel, Switzerland.)

M2-channel blockers

Amantadine was the first of the M2-channel blockers, with a main indication for the treatment of Parkinson's disease; however, it was licensed for the treatment and prophylaxis of influenza in 1966. The licence was strain-specific until 1977 pending the accumulation of data on sensitivity to a wider range of viruses covering the period from 1935 to 1977, when a general licence was granted for influenza A. The initial dosage was 100 mg twice daily, but this has since been reduced to 100 mg daily for use against influenza in some countries, which has significantly improved the side-effect profile of the drug. Rimantadine is a newer drug of the same class with an identical mode of action. The two drugs are considered indistinguishable in terms of their effectiveness for treatment and prophylaxis, but rimantadine is associated with fewer side-effects on the central nervous system (CNS). Both drugs must be given as soon as possible after the onset of symptoms (within 48 h of symptom onset/exposure for treatment and prophylaxis, respectively). Because influenza B does not contain an M2-ion channel, neither drug is effective against this virus, but this limitation is not relevant to pandemic preparedness.

Many studies have demonstrated that the M2-channel blockers are efficacious for the treatment and prophylaxis of influenza. Over 80 clinical trials and observational studies on amantadine can be found in the literature, involving over 19,000 patients ranging in age from children (>1 year) to the very elderly (up to 99 years), though the drug is not licensed in children under 10 years of age. Specific settings for these studies have included healthy volunteers, hospital staff, primary care patients, prisons, military personnel and residential homes for the elderly and learning disabled.

Treatment efficacy/effectiveness

In general, amantadine has been reported to be effective in reducing respiratory symptoms and the duration of fever. In healthy adults (aged 18–64 years) the reduction in duration of fever is reported to be 1.0–1.5 days. Similar data are available in the elderly and small numbers of older children; however, very few data exist regarding use in patients with high-risk conditions. A very small number of studies have reported a reduction in secondary complications, but the vast majority of these patients were healthy military personnel; most studies have not assessed whether the M2-channel blockers reduce complications.

Efficacy/effectiveness for prophylaxis

A Cochrane review (updated 2008) concluded that in healthy adults, the effectiveness of both drugs for the prevention of influenza (used to prevent clinical influenza) was 25% and the efficacy (used to prevent serologically confirmed influenza) was 61%. In the elderly, the majority of data on prophylaxis originate from use in outbreaks, where effectiveness has ranged from 37–80% in mainly vaccinated populations.

Adverse events

The most common side-effects reported with the use of M2-channel blockers involve the CNS: anxiety, difficulty in concentrating, insomnia, dizziness, headache and jitteriness. In elderly subjects additional manifestations include confusion, disorientation, mood and memory alteration, nightmares, ataxia, tremors, acute psychosis, delirium and hallucinations. Gastrointestinal and cardiovascular side-effects have also been reported.

J. Van-Tam and R.K. Gupta

In general the incidence of side-effects is proportional to age, being 15–30% in healthy adults and 31% in the elderly (9% CNS side-effects) when given at 200 mg daily. The incidence of side-effects associated with the lower dose of 100 mg daily is, however, likely to be somewhat lower (but not zero) and might be reduced further by intermittent daily dosing in the elderly (100 mg at intervals of >1 day). In order to avoid accumulation and an increased risk of side-effects, dose adjustment should be made in patients with a significant degree of renal impairment.

Resistance

Perhaps the biggest concern about the M2-channel blockers in relation to their potential utility as pandemic agents is the emergence of resistance. There are numerous reports in the literature which document the rapid emergence of resistant viruses (within days) after the instigation of therapy; in general this occurs more commonly when the drug is used simultaneously for treatment and prophylaxis in the same setting. Of greater concern is the fact that such viruses appear transmissible and of equivalent virulence to sensitive strains, thus the emergence of resistance does not confer a survival disadvantage to the virus.

Aside from reports of the emergence of resistant viruses under pressure from drug usage, routine surveillance of laboratory isolates of influenza suggest that historically the prevalence of adamantine-resistant viruses has been low (<1%) Since about 2000, however, this proportion has risen sharply, especially with respect to A/H3N2 viruses. By 2006, levels of resistance in A/H3N2 viruses had reached 75% in China, 70% in Hong Kong and about 90% in the USA, prompting the US Centers for Disease Control and Prevention to warn against the use of amantadine and rimantadine for treatment or prevention of seasonal influenza A.

With regard to influenza A/H5N1, of the four major clades or sub-clades associated with human disease (1, 2.1, 2.2 and 2.3), 100% of clade 1 viruses and at least 80% of clade 2.1 viruses are already resistant to amantadine and rimantadine. Resistant A/H7 and A/H9 viruses have also been identified. This is a necessary consideration given the potential pandemic threat posed by A/H5N1 and other avian viruses, although it must be stressed again that the identity of the next pandemic subtype remains unknown.

Neuraminidase inhibitors

The story of the development of neuraminidase inhibitors begins with the discovery of neuraminidase on the surface of the influenza virus in 1942. In 1969 Meindl and Tuppy described DANA (2-deoxy-2,3-dehydro-N-acetylneuraminic acid) – a sialic acid analogue capable of inhibiting neuraminidase. In 1976, an analogue, FANA (2-deoxy-2,3-dehydro-N-trifluoroacetylneuraminic acid), was shown to prevent the replication of influenza virus *in vitro*. However, neither DANA nor FANA possessed the correct pharmacokinetic properties to be effective therapeutic agents in man, due to rapid elimination from the body. In 1983 the crystal structure of influenza neuraminidase was described allowing DANA to be modified by rational computer-aided design. This work ultimately led to the discovery of zanamivir, followed shortly by oseltamivir.

Zanamivir (Relenza®) and oseltamivir (Tamiflu®) were both licensed in 1999. Both molecules bind to a highly conserved site on the neuraminidase and are highly selective for influenza virus neuraminidase, which strongly reduces the chances of side-effects due to the inadvertent inhibition of human enzyme systems. The main ingredient in Tamiflu is the pro-drug oseltamivir phosphate, which is converted into its active form (oseltamivir carboxylate) once ingested.

Pharmacokinetic differences between zanamivir and oseltamivir

Zanamivir is delivered as a dry powder by oral inhalation through a purposely designed Diskhaler® device, because it is extremely poorly bioavailable via the gastrointestinal tract (<5%). Even when administered by oral inhalation it is relatively poorly bioavailable (10–20%). Scintography shows that 77% of a 10 mg dose is deposited in the oropharynx, 1% in the trachea and 13% in the lungs. Thus drug levels in the respiratory mucosa, at the site of virus replication, are relatively high, but patients are not systemically exposed to the drug to any great extent. Zanamivir is excreted almost unchanged in the urine, but because of its wide safety margins, no dose adjustment is necessary in renal impairment. In contrast, oseltamivir is 75% bioavailable by oral administration. It is systemically absorbed and achieves therapeutic levels in many tissues. It is extensively converted by enzymes in the liver into the active form and thereafter excreted via the kidneys. Some dose adjustment is necessary in severe renal failure. Both zanamivir and oseltamivir have relatively short serum half-lives, necessitating twice daily administration for treatment.

Treatment efficacy/effectiveness

The clinical trials programmes of both neuraminidase inhibitors have been aimed at gaining licensure for efficacy in treating influenza – inevitably this has meant that those trials have assessed major symptoms as the primary endpoint. While this was clearly necessary for commercialization, an unfortunate consequence is that relatively few primary data are available on outcomes of public health significance (e.g. hospitalization and mortality), which have considerable relevance to pandemic stockpiling decisions. Another inevitable and unavoidable drawback in the data relates to the fact that the clinical trials have been performed in the setting of 'normal' seasonal influenza (A/H3N2, A/H1N1 and B); it is arguable that these viruses produce milder disease than might be encountered with a future pandemic virus. This problem is insurmountable and emphasizes the need to have systems in place in advance of the next pandemic for the rapid assessment of the effectiveness of antiviral drugs (and vaccines).

In the major clinical trials of zanamivir, a median 1.5 day reduction in duration of major symptoms (headache, myalgia, sore throat, cough, fever or feverishness) was obtained in adults and children. This was the case whether patients with influenza symptoms were considered or just those with laboratory-confirmed influenza. Return to normal activities was attained 1.75–2.0 days earlier. Of relevance to a possible secondary public health benefit during a pandemic was the fact that zanamivir

J. Van-Tam and R.K. Gupta

reduced virus shedding in deliberately infected volunteers by 96% compared with placebo, thus infectiousness to others should also be reduced as a result of treating the individual. The pooled results from seven double-blind placebo-controlled trials of zanamivir suggest a significant 20–25% reduction in complications requiring the use of antibiotics associated with zanamivir treatment, which was most pronounced for lower respiratory tract illness.

Oseltamivir treatment produces clinical benefits that are highly similar to those for zanamivir, with an average reduction in the duration of major symptoms of 1.0–1.5 days compared with placebo in adults and children. Similar data are also available on the reduction of virus shedding. In an analysis of over 3500 patients across ten clinical trials, oseltamivir significantly reduced lower respiratory tract complications requiring antibiotics by 55%, pneumonia by 61% and hospitalizations by 59% (50% in high-risk patients). A smaller study in children also revealed that oseltamivir significantly reduced all complications by 40% and antibiotic usage by 24%. More recent data, mainly from observational studies, have confirmed the effect of oseltamivir in reducing hospitalizations and pneumonia. One study has now suggested that oseltamivir produced a 70% reduction in mortality in hospitalized adults.

Finally, limited information is available on the effectiveness of oseltamivir against human A/H5N1 disease. Data have been presented on 188 confirmed cases of A/H5N1 treated with oseltamivir and 56 untreated patients. The virus infections came from clades 1, 2.1 and 2.2, and the interval between symptom onset and treatment initiation was variable. Most treatment doses were standard. Survival was significantly higher among treated versus untreated patients (47% versus 12%), although this is still only modest. These data may not be strictly relevant to pandemic influenza since: (i) the origin of the next pandemic virus is unknown; and (ii) A/H5N1 is presently an avian virus that is non-adapted to man.

Efficacy/effectiveness for prophylaxis

Zanamivir and oseltamivir have both been assessed for long-term prophylaxis (up to 28 and 42 days, respectively) and short-term post-exposure prophylaxis (PEP). Zanamivir was evaluated in two studies of long-term prophylaxis, with an efficacy of 67% against laboratory-confirmed influenza A in one study and 83% in the other. With regard to short-term PEP, data are available from two household PEP studies which demonstrated 80% efficacy in reducing the chances of another influenza case in the household.

More comprehensive data on prophylaxis are available for oseltamivir. Regarding long-term prophylaxis in adults and the frail elderly, effectiveness (intention-to-treat analysis) of 76% and 92%, respectively, has been reported. Of greater importance are the data from two large trials of household PEP, which reveal an effectiveness of 92% and 63%, respectively.

The available evidence suggests that when either drug is used for treatment or short-term PEP, antibody may still be formed as a response to influenza infection, even in patients who remain asymptomatic. This is especially relevant given the current interest in using neuraminidase inhibitors for household PEP during a pandemic (in addition to treatment of the index case).

Adverse events and drug interactions

In clinical trials of zanamivir, the incidence of side-effects was slightly higher in the placebo groups than in the treatment groups (38% versus 33%). All of these were symptoms normally encountered with influenza (e.g. nasal symptoms, diarrhoea, nausea, headache, cough), suggesting that genuine symptoms were reported as adverse events. The only genuine issue that has arisen with zanamivir is the possibility of induced bronchospasm (sometimes severe) in a small proportion of patients, not necessarily those with underlying lung disease. Because zanamivir is poorly bio-available the potential for drug interactions is extremely low. Dose adjustment in patients with renal dysfunction is not necessary.

The main side-effects encountered with oseltamivir are gastrointestinal, typically nausea and vomiting. The incidence of these side-effects is about 10% (each) at treatment dose, but severity can be reduced by taking drug with food and tends to diminish after the first few doses. Few other adverse events are reported. In 2006 the Japanese regulatory authorities issued a warning in relation to the possibility of sudden self-injury or confusion after several reports came to light of teenagers recently treated with oseltamivir, including three deaths that may have been suicides. Oseltamivir requires dose adjustment in severe renal impairment.

Neither zanamivir nor oseltamivir is licensed for use during pregnancy and lactation. Full data on side-effects, interactions, contraindications and safety warnings for amantadine, zanamivir and oseltamivir can be found by consulting the relevant Summary of Product Characteristics.

Resistance

Resistance to zanamivir is hardly described and so far resistant viruses appear less virulent than wild-type viruses. Historically, since launch, the level of resistance reported with oseltamivir has also been low, with resistant viruses being less fit and accounting for <1% of viruses in adults and about 4% in children. Some Japanese data reported rates of up to 18% in children treated with oseltamivir, however, this may have been due to under-dosing, specific to how the drug was used in Japan.

In the 2007–2008 northern hemisphere winter season, an influenza A/H1N1 virus circulated widely in Europe. A subpopulation of viruses contained a mutation in the neuraminidase gene denoted H274Y (substitution of tyrosine for histidine at amino acid position 274) which, when present on the N1 neuraminidase moiety, was consistent with very high-level resistance to oseltamivir. The proportion of resistant viruses varied widely from country to country, ranging from 67% to zero. In the following season (2008–2009) although the northern hemisphere winter season was dominated by an A/H3N2 epidemic, the A/H1N1 viruses in circulation in many parts of the world often carried the H274Y mutation. It has become clear that these viruses also carry additional co-mutations in the neuraminidase gene which appear to allow the introduction of H274Y without any detrimental impact on fitness *in vivo*, i.e. the virus remains pathogenic and transmissible. The important features of this phenomenon can be summarized as:

- The H274Y mutation produces changes in the N1 protein that result in high-level resistance to oseltamivir.
- It is too early to say if A/H1N1 oseltamivir-resistant viruses will remain dominant or even continue to circulate in the long term.
- The resistance conferred by the H274Y mutation cannot be overcome by increasing treatment dosage.
- Resistance did not arise due to treatment pressure; most cases from which resistant virus was recovered had not been treated with oseltamivir.
- The resistant virus is pathogenic and transmissible but does not produce clinical disease that is obviously more or less severe than that occurring with sensitive A/H1N1 viruses.
- These viruses remain susceptible to zanamivir.

At this stage, the implications of this mutation for pandemic stockpiling of neuraminidase inhibitors are not clear and the situation requires close monitoring. A/H5N1 viruses carrying the H274Y mutation have been reported in small numbers, but A/H5N1 may or may not be the cause of the next pandemic. The H274Y mutation does not produce oseltamivir resistance in non-N1 viruses.

The other two well-described mutations associated with oseltamivir resistance are denoted R292K (produces reduced susceptibility to oseltamivir in N2-containing viruses) and E119V (affecting N2- or N9-containing viruses).

The emergence of oseltamivir resistance against seasonal influenza reinforces the need to take a risk-averse approach and consider a mixed stockpile of both oseltamivir and zanamivir so that options are still available in the event of one drug failing. It also reinforces the need for layered containment approaches to pandemic preparedness (Chapter 10), so that undue reliance is not placed on one single intervention.

Ease of use and suitability for pandemic deployment

Zanamivir suffers from three possible drawbacks compared with oseltamivir, regarding ease of use and mass deployment. First, it is an orally inhaled product that requires the use of a Diskhaler® device. One study has raised questions about whether this device can be managed by the elderly or people with poor hand strength/coordination; however, the manufacturers have produced opposing data. Second, it must be used cautiously in people with asthma and other chronic pulmonary diseases, and third, it is not licensed for children less than 5 years of age.

In contrast, oseltamivir is licensed from 1 year of age upwards, is given orally by capsule and a paediatric suspension is also available. However, the reports from Japan of confusion and self-injury in adolescents mean that diligence is needed when using the drug in this age group until the picture is clearer.

Of definite relevance to pandemic stockpiling is the fact that oseltamivir is available to governments (only) in magistral formulation. The active pharmaceutical ingredient is a water-soluble dry powder, with a very long shelf-life (many years) when stored in sealed drums (Fig. 8.2). When dissolved in water (15 mg/ml) the solution is stable for 3 weeks at 25°C and for 6 weeks at 5°C. For countries with fewer available resources for procurement, the magistral formulation provides a lower-cost stockpiling option. Of course, this strategy is pointless unless the pharmacy infrastructure

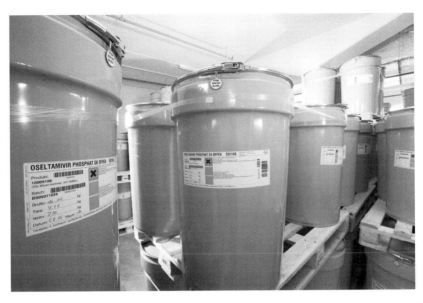

Fig. 8.2. Oseltamivir active pharmaceutical ingredient in sealed barrels. (Kindly supplied by F. Hoffman-La Roche Ltd, Basel, Switzerland.)

within the country is sufficient to cope with large-scale reconstitution in the event of a pandemic. The reconstituted mixture is also foul-tasting and this needs to be taken into consideration, especially regarding use in young children where a masking flavour is likely to be needed. A comparison of the main features of zanamivir and oseltamivir is provided in Table 8.2.

Practicalities relating to stockpiling

For the first time ever, antiviral drugs will be available to counter the effects of the next pandemic. While it is clear that pandemic vaccine will not be available for several months, it is equally clear that unless antiviral drugs are stockpiled in advance, there will be insufficient supplies. With regard to pandemic stockpiling, this must always be undertaken against a background of considerable uncertainty about the origin of the next pandemic virus. In this regard it is reassuring that *in vitro* data are available on the efficacy of both neuraminidase inhibitors against representative viruses covering all nine neuraminidases, including A/H1N1, A/H1N9, A/H2N2, A/H2N3, A/H3N2, A/H4N6, A/H8N4, A/H5N1, A/H3N8, A/H10N7, A/H12N5, A/H7N7 and A/H9N2. Thus the first question is answered about the broad activity of neuraminidase inhibitors (all known N types) and the likelihood of having some activity against the next pandemic virus. The data pertaining to clinical benefits and reductions in complications have all been obtained in the setting of seasonal influenza. It is not clear if these benefits can be translated into effects against a novel pandemic virus, although likely to be the case to some extent. Nevertheless, this question simply cannot be answered in advance and ultimately it necessary to accept or reject this inherent risk. If antiviral drugs are to be considered, the most important

Table 8.2. Comparison of the main features of zanamivir and oseltamivir.

Feature	Zanamivir (Relenza®)	Oseltamivir (Tamiflu®)
Formulations	Dry powder for oral inhalation	Dry powder in capsules; paediatric suspension; magistral
Age range	≥5 years	≥1 year
Data on treatment efficacy	Yes	Yes
Data on short-term PEP	Yes	Yes
Data on long-term prophylaxis	Yes	Yes
Drug interactions	Low	Low
Side-effects	Mainly respiratory	Mainly gastrointestinal
Warnings	Bronchospasm	Self-harm and confusion (Japanese data only)
Bioavailability	10–20%	75%
Treatment dosage	Twice daily (5 days)	Twice daily (5 days)
PEP dosage	Once daily (10 days)	Once daily (10 days)
Long-term prophylaxis dosage	Once daily (up to 28 days)	Once daily (up to 42 days)
Dose adjustment in renal failure	No	Yes (in severe renal failure)
Licensed in pregnancy and lactation	No	No
Significant resistance to date	No	Yes (but A/H1N1 only)

PEP, post-exposure prophylaxis.

questions then relate to their deployment strategy. In practical terms, this can be considered at various levels according to the desired public health objectives. Potential pandemic deployment strategies for antiviral drugs are summarized in Table 8.3.

It is not possible to specify for individual countries whether antivirals should be procured and how they should be deployed. There is no 'one size fits all' approach and what can be achieved depends to a large extent on what can be afforded, governmental priorities and pandemic risk assessment. The larger the stockpile, the greater the options that can be considered for strategic use. Given what is known about previous clinical attack rates in pandemics of the 20th century, a stockpile of around 40% of population size is needed before a 'treat-all' strategy can be achieved in practice (unless the clinical attack rate is very low); and at least 60–70% would be needed to be able to consider a strategy of 'treatment + household PEP'.

Rapid delivery and wastage

Data obtained from an open-label study of oseltamivir clearly show that the reduction in illness duration was 3.1 days when treatment was initiated 12 h after symptom onset, compared with at 48 h. These data illustrate the point that maximum clinical benefit for the individual is conferred by rapid treatment. Similarly, since virus shedding is maximal soon after symptom onset, early treatment also reduces infectiousness. Modelling data suggest that, at a population level, initiation of therapy (whether treatment only for individuals or treatment + household PEP) within 12–24 h will be vital in maximizing public health benefits.

Table 8.3. Possible pandemic deployment strategies for antiviral drugs.

Public health objective	Deployment strategy				
	Treatment only for selected groups based on high-risk status[a]	Treatment only for selected groups based on employment category/importance of pandemic role[b]	Treatment only for whole population[c]	Treatment for whole population plus household PEP	Long-term prophylaxis for selected groups based on employment category/importance of pandemic role[d]
Reduce overall mortality and complications	✓		✓✓	✓✓	
Reduce symptoms and increase speed of return to normal activity	✓	✓	✓	✓	
Slow rate of occurrence of new cases and make pandemic's impact flatter and longer (reduce peak incidence), making it easier to cope with			✓	✓✓	
Reduce infectiousness and prevent secondary cases occurring			✓	✓✓	
Prevent cases almost completely in some groups					✓
Reduce impact on CNI and 'essential services'		✓	✓	✓✓	✓✓✓
Relative quantity of drugs needed	Medium/large	Small/medium	Very large	Extremely large	Medium/large

PEP, post-exposure prophylaxis; CNI, critical national infrastructure.
[a]High-risk groups will not be known until after the pandemic starts and their identification will depend on high-quality clinico-epidemiological data.
[b]Treating selected subgroups will depend upon public, political and ethical acceptability (regarding those excluded).
[c]Secondary benefits from 'whole population' strategies depend upon rapid institution of therapy after onset of symptoms (in index case) and adequate logistics.
[d]Long-term prophylaxis for selected groups depends upon continuing therapy until pandemic vaccine can be given (i.e. rarely practical).

J. Van-Tam and R.K. Gupta

Focus Box 8.1. What does modelling tell us about antiviral usage?

P.G. Grove, Senior Principal Analyst, Department of Health, Health Protection Analytical Team

Antiviral drugs could be used for universal pre-exposure (long-term) prophylaxis. This would be a very effective approach as the reduction in transmission, combined with the protective nature of the antiviral, would mean that there would be only a handful of cases throughout the period of prophylaxis. However, for a country like the UK the amount of antiviral required would be astronomical, at around 45 million treatment courses per week. When the stockpile became exhausted then the national epidemic would take off exactly as if there had been no prophylaxis, except delayed by a little longer, perhaps twice the period of prophylaxis.

Antiviral drugs could more usefully be used for the treatment of all those with symptoms. This could be combined with post-exposure prophylaxis of household contacts (also described as household prophylaxis). Individual antiviral treatment is known to reduce the duration and severity of seasonal influenza as well as the occurrence of secondary complications and could have some effect on the overall attack rate (possibly a 5–10% reduction), although there would probably be a greater effect on the peak incidence. However, the household prophylaxis approach can also significantly reduce the number of cases and hence further reduce the number of severe cases and deaths.

If combined with school closures, the household prophylaxis approach could reduce the attack rate by one-third with perhaps a two-thirds reduction in peak incidence. Estimates of the impact of both treatment and household prophylaxis need to take account of the fact that symptoms will arise about 1 day after infection and it might take 1–2 days for the antivirals to be administered. The effectiveness of antivirals in reducing transmission is greatly reduced if mechanisms do not exist to ensure treatment within 1 day of symptoms arising in a patient.

Antivirals can also be used in a more aggressive approach to contain a pandemic 'at source'. An extensive prophylaxis policy based on targeting the people closest to the first few cases (up to perhaps 50,000 'contacts' in a town), combined with stringent social distance measures and the use of area quarantine, could contain an outbreak with, perhaps, three million courses of antivirals. Even if the strategy fails to contain the disease, it might delay its progress by around a month. This concept has been adopted by the World Health Organization. However, the practical difficulties of implementing the strategy are enormous and it is best adapted to rural communities where the rigorous social distance measures and area quarantine may be possible. In this approach the pandemic strain is eradicated having infected no more than a few tens of people and hence early detection of the 'first few cases' is essential.

Similar modelling for the UK, assuming that the pandemic originates outside the country with multiple cases coming in from abroad, indicates that even with the more practical (for the UK) measures of, say, prophylaxis of all those within 5 km of a case together with 90% school and 50% workplace closures, containment requires impractically large antiviral stockpiles. All these interventions will have knock-on wider societal effects as people stay away from workplaces.

Thus, the decision to stockpile antiviral drugs carries with it the necessity to plan a strategy for effective, timely delivery. This needs to take into account the availability of medical and pharmacy staff and the legal basis of prescribing (which may require alteration for a pandemic). If rapid delivery at population level cannot be achieved through conventional physician prescribing, it may be necessary to consider allowing prescribing by non-physician healthcare workers or the use of protocol-driven 'prescribing' by non-healthcare personnel. For example, the UK is planning to deliver antiviral drugs via a specific national telephone helpline, using protocol-based 'prescribing' by non-healthcare workers and collection from specified 'local collection points' by a friend or relative. One frequently mentioned option is the pre-issue of antivirals, in effect 'home stockpiling'. Although often quoted, there are a variety of reasons why this is not a good idea:

- The national stockpile would automatically have to be >100% of population size on equity grounds (it cannot be predicted in advance who will get pandemic influenza and who will not).
- Stocks could not be moved around the country to where they are most needed.
- There is likely to be early use and exhaustion of stocks as untrained people use the drug too early.
- The likelihood of early development of antiviral resistance may increase.

It is almost inevitable that antiviral drugs will need to be administered without diagnostic confirmation of any sort, partly because this service will not be available in sufficient capacity during a pandemic, and partly because the emphasis will be on rapid delivery and waiting for diagnostic tests will result in unacceptable delays. Thus a case definition will be required and real-time epidemiological data will be needed to optimize its sensitivity and specificity. Nevertheless, wastage (treating people who do not have pandemic influenza) is an inevitable consequence of mass population-level deployment. It must simply be factored into considerations of stockpile size and the logistic planning of mass treatment.

Choice of antiviral drugs for stockpiling

Although amantadine and rimantadine may be up to ten times cheaper than the neuraminidase inhibitors, these drugs do not constitute rational choices for stockpiling; at most they should be held in very small quantities. The CNS side-effect profile of the M2-channel blockers (especially amantadine) is unacceptable compared with the neuraminidase inhibitors and there are too many concerns about the rapid emergence of transmissible resistant viruses. Zanamivir in one sense offers the most promise in relation to the lowest likelihood of the emergence of resistance, but is handicapped by its relatively cumbersome mode of delivery and its licence, which does not cover pre-school children. Oseltamivir is the obvious choice in relation to its ease of use, but concerns exist about the emergence of resistance associated with a specific mutation that can affect N1-containing viruses.

Notwithstanding, the phenomenon of antiviral resistance should be placed in context. If a virus is fully resistant to a given drug by the time it enters a country, then, to all intents and purposes, the drug will be ineffective. However, if only a small proportion of viruses are initially resistant or if resistance emerges for the first time within-country, then modelling data suggest that the public health value of mass treatment (with or without household PEP) will be only modestly diminished.

Given that no one drug is ideal, it makes sense to aim for a mixed stockpile, which comprises both zanamivir and oseltamivir and allows the pursuit of a secondary strategy objective should one drug fail in practice. It is also necessary to plan rational alternative strategies of use should this circumstance arise; for example, limiting treatment to certain patient subgroups. Figure 8.3 illustrates what is in the public domain about national stockpiling of neuraminidase inhibitors at the present time. For ease of comparison, it depicts the relative size of stockpiles in relation to the proportion of the host population that could be treated. However, individual countries represented may not pursue such a strategy.

8.3   Antibiotics

The link between influenza A and secondary bacterial infection is well established. Many studies have demonstrated a temporal relationship between seasonal influenza activity and bacterial pneumonia, and this association is also true for all three pandemics of the 20th century, in which substantial morbidity and mortality were attributed to bacterial complications.

It is an attractive suggestion that if antiviral drugs 'treat' pandemic influenza effectively and quickly their success will be such that bacterial complications requiring antibiotic treatment will be rare. However, this is a relatively unsafe planning assumption because, as discussed earlier, the evidence that neuraminidase inhibitors reduce the likelihood of bacterial complications is derived from usage during seasonal influenza rather than pandemic influenza. In addition, it is clear that pandemic vaccine will not be available for several months (Chapter 9). Thus it is a reasonable assumption that bacterial complications of influenza will occur and require consideration as part of overall pandemic preparedness. The sheer number of influenza cases coupled with disproportionate effects on the elderly and those with chronic diseases is likely to lead to large numbers of patients with secondary pneumonia, of whom a proportion will have an associated bacteraemia. Furthermore, the burden of disease is likely to be even greater in developing nations where bacterial pneumonia is more common, and where immune deficiency, for example due to HIV/AIDS, is more prevalent. Patients with bacterial pneumonia complicating influenza may be more likely to require medical attention and hospital care than most patients with uncomplicated primary influenza infection.

The projected demand for antibiotics therefore warrants consideration of methods to increase stocks of key agents as part of pandemic preparedness efforts. While the effect that antiviral drugs will have on pandemic case fatality rate will remain unknown until such drugs are first used against the emergent virus, the effectiveness of antibiotics against bacterial pneumonia and bacteraemia is much easier to predict through current everyday experience of use in routine clinical practice, however, it is accepted that new resistance could emerge. Modelling data suggest that although antibiotics would have zero impact on the incidence of influenza (having no action against a viral agent), as many deaths might be averted through appropriate use of antibiotics as through the use of antiviral drugs.

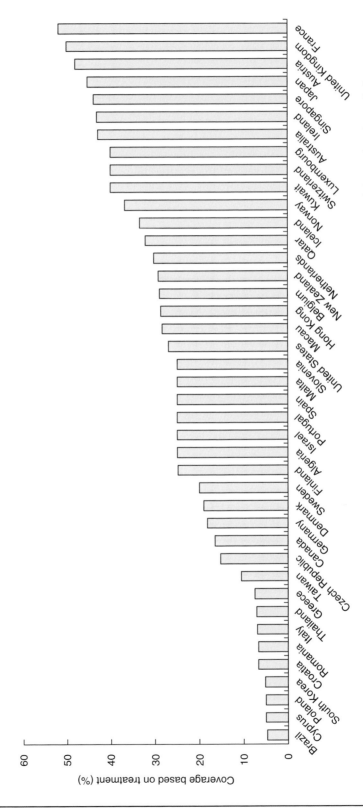

Fig. 8.3. Public domain antiviral stockpiles by country, January 2009, as ability to treat indicated percentage of the national population (although the treatment strategy may not necessarily be chosen by each country). (Kindly supplied by F. Hoffman-La Roche Ltd, Basel, Switzerland.) Sources: media/national pandemic plans (last updated Jan. 2009) and population figures from http://www.geottive.com (as of Jan. 2007).

J. Van-Tam and R.K. Gupta

What size of stockpile is needed?

One critical issue for governments is therefore what quantity of antibiotics to stockpile. In terms of estimating the overall stockpile size required, the proportion of pandemic influenza cases that will progress to bacterial complications needs to be estimated. The difficulty in making such an estimate relates partly to the paucity of contemporary data that specifically describe the incidence of bacterial complications after influenza and partly to the fact that widespread use of neuraminidase inhibitors, rarely used for seasonal influenza, might reduce the development of antimicrobial drug-related complications by 25–40%, but this is far from certain. Data from the three pandemics of the 20th century suggest that bacterial pneumonia developed in 15–20% of influenza patients; however, some estimates for seasonal influenza are far higher than this.

Placing these data in the context of a population clinical attack rate in the range of 25–50%, we can estimate that an antimicrobial drug stockpile is likely to be needed for a minimum of 10% of the population. This figure does not account for wastage, misdiagnosis (if, as is most likely, prescribing is empirical, based on clinical suspicion alone and unsupported by bacteriology investigations) or a higher rate of secondary bacterial complication than expected. It is also based on a strategy of treatment only. This is also questionable since during a pandemic certain patient groups, such as those with chronic obstructive pulmonary disease, might well benefit from prophylactic antibiotics given with an antiviral drug at the onset of influenza-like illness; such a strategy would potentially reduce demand for repeat consultations in high-risk patients. The rationale for this prescribing strategy is further strengthened by anticipating a shortage of hospital capacity compared with the demand for treatment of established pneumonia.

Which antibiotics should be stockpiled?

Clinical management guidelines for pandemic influenza exist in relatively few countries but have recommended co-amoxiclav (amoxicillin + clavulanate) or doxycycline, third-generation cephalosporins or respiratory fluoroquinolones, and second-generation cephalosporins, macrolides or co-trimoxazole as first-line empirical antibiotic choices for community-acquired pneumonia associated with pandemic influenza. The recent emergence of community-acquired MRSA (methicillin-resistant *Staphylococcus aureus*) has raised fears that this could be a significant pathogen in relation to a future pandemic. If so, stocks of vancomycin, linezolid, quinopristin/dalfopristin and tigecycline would also come under consideration.

The example of MRSA highlights a need for the exact make-up of antibiotic stocks to reflect the prevalent organisms and their antimicrobial sensitivities. Real-time surveillance of the bacteria most commonly isolated from the human respiratory tract during community-acquired pneumonia, namely *Streptococcus pneumoniae*, *Haemophilus influenzae* and *S. aureus*, would enable recommendation of antimicrobial drugs on the basis of the proportion of respiratory tract isolates likely to be susceptible at a particular point in time. For example, it is known in the UK that most MRSA isolates are sensitive to doxycycline, rifampicin (rifampin) and to a lesser extent trimethoprim. Less severe MRSA infections treated with these widely available and inexpensive drugs would be expected to respond. Finally, a surveillance programme may also provide early warning of likely clinical failures caused by emerging resistance.

Use of existing ciprofloxacin stockpiles

A number of countries hold stockpiles of ciprofloxacin as a bioterrorism countermeasure. Data from the UK suggest that this quinolone can be expected to be active against most *H. influenzae* and *S. aureus* isolates, as well as atypical organisms. However, ciprofloxacin's activity against *S. pneumoniae* is only intermediate, and a significant number of bacterial pneumonias complicating influenza may not respond to empirical treatment with this agent. Therefore, in a pandemic, empirical ciprofloxacin use could be justified only if all other more suitable antimicrobial drug supplies were exhausted. Additionally, ciprofloxacin could be targeted during a pandemic to persons previously vaccinated against pneumococcal infection who did not have signs of clinical severity. Theoretical support for this approach comes from the USA, where use of a seven-valent conjugate vaccine since 2000 has resulted in declining invasive pneumococcal disease, and relatively infrequent influenza-related deaths caused by pneumococci in children.

Size, storage and turnover of stockpiles

Decisions regarding the composition of pandemic stockpiles, procurements and size depend primarily on financial considerations at a national level, although international organizations may have influence through a variety of mechanisms, from direct financial support to centralized antibiotic stockpiling. The initial stockpile needs not only to be purchased and stored, but also maintained, potentially over a significant time period. Vaccines for influenza virus subtype A/H5N1 and neuraminidase inhibitors are being stockpiled exclusively for pre-pandemic and pandemic use. By contrast, antimicrobial drugs are widely used every day, and therefore stockpiling as part of pandemic preparedness requires a different approach.

This difference means that antimicrobial drugs could act as a buffer stock (conceptually similar to vendor-managed inventory) in most healthcare systems, rather than a true stockpile. Increased stores of antimicrobial drugs could be channelled into day-to-day use and replaced through fresh procurement. Thus, over time, the amount, proportion and range of these agents held can be slowly altered. This ongoing process of continual interpandemic use and restocking make such a 'stockpile' far less vulnerable than antiviral drugs to exceed expiry dates and far more responsive to changes in antimicrobial drug sensitivity detected between the date of procurement and the onset of the next pandemic. Effective storage of such buffer stocks could also be facilitated; whereas antiviral drugs and vaccines essentially need to be held in secure centralized storage (the latter within the cold chain) until eventual deployment, antimicrobial drugs can be held, at least in part, lower down the supply chain by wholesalers and community pharmacies or their equivalent. This would expedite local delivery during a pandemic when services and transport links may be compromised.

8.4 Summary

Modern influenza antiviral drugs – the neuraminidase inhibitors – have an important potential role in pandemic preparedness. These would need to be stockpiled in advance to ensure availability. It cannot be known in advance of the emergence of the next pandemic how effective these drugs will be, but significant effects on morbidity (complications) and illness severity seem likely and mortality may also be reduced. Effective deployment will depend on careful consideration of the desired public health objective and matching this to an appropriate 'treatment' strategy. Faulty logistic plans and delays in initiation of treatment will compromise the effectiveness of any programme. It is not possible to predict in advance whether resistance will emerge as a major problem; a mixed stockpile of zanamivir and oseltamivir therefore seems prudent.

Bacterial pneumonia is likely to be an important cause of morbidity and mortality during the next pandemic. In many countries, pandemic preparedness activities have so far overlooked or given insufficient emphasis and priority to antibiotic stockpiling especially because as many lives may be saved by use of antibiotics as by antiviral drugs. In most modern healthcare systems, which increasingly emphasize just-in-time supply chains, shortages of antimicrobial drugs may occur rapidly unless more are stockpiled. Buffer stock management at a local level, informed by antimicrobial sensitivity data, should enable appropriate, usable stocks to be available in the event of a pandemic. Increased global production of high-quality generic antibiotics is also needed, along with appropriate national storage and delivery mechanisms.

8.5 Summary Points

- M2-channel blockers and the newer neuraminidase inhibitors (zanamivir and oseltamivir) are available for the treatment of influenza. Neuraminidase inhibitors are vastly superior and have far fewer side-effects.
- Although the effectiveness of neuraminidase inhibitors against a future pandemic virus cannot be known in advance, there is a good chance that these drugs will be active across all nine neuraminidases and that they will reduce both the duration of symptoms and the rate of complications and hospitalizations. It is not known if they will reduce the case fatality rate, but this is not ruled out.
- A mixed stockpile of neuraminidase inhibitors is recommended.
- Antibiotics should be stockpiled in anticipation of secondary bacterial complications in 15–20% of pandemic influenza cases.
- The stockpiled antibiotic agents should offer broad cover against *S. pneumoniae*, *S. aureus* and *H. influenzae* when used empirically.

Further Reading

Antiviral drugs

Aoki, F.Y., Macleod, M.D., Paggiaro, P., Carewicz, O., El Sawy, A., Wat, C., Griffiths, M., Waalberg, E. and Ward, P.; IMPACT Study Group (2003) Early administration of oral oseltamivir increases the benefits of influenza treatment. *Journal of Antimicrobial Chemotherapy* 51, 123–129.

Cheer, S.M. and Wagstaff, A.J. (2002) Zanamivir: an update of its use in influenza. *Drugs* 62, 71–106.

Dunn, C.J. and Goa, K.L. (1999) Zanamivir: a review of its use in influenza. *Drugs* 58, 761–784.

Electronic Medicines Compendium (2008) *Summary of Product Characteristics: Relenza®* *(zanamivir) 5 mg/dose inhalation powder.* http://emc.medicines.org.uk/document. aspx?documentId=2608 (accessed May 2009).

Electronic Medicines Compendium (2009) *Summary of Product Characteristics: Tamiflu®* *(oseltamivir) 75 mg hard capsule.* http://emc.medicines.org.uk/medicine/10446/SPC/ Tamiflu+75mg+hard+capsule/ (accessed May 2009).

Ferguson, N.M., Cummings, D.A., Fraser, C., Cajka, J.C., Cooley, P.C. and Burke, D.S. (2005) Strategies for containing an emerging influenza pandemic in Southeast Asia. *Nature* 437, 209–214.

Kaiser, L., Wat, C., Mills, T., Mahoney, P., Ward, P. and Hayden, F. (2003) Impact of oseltamivir treatment on influenza-related lower respiratory tract complications and hospitalizations. *Archives of Internal Medicine* 163, 1667–1672.

Ward, P., Small, I., Smith, J., Suter, P. and Dutkowski, R. (2005) Oseltamivir (Tamiflu) and its potential use in the event of an influenza pandemic. *Journal of Antimicrobial Chemotherapy* 55(Suppl. S1), i5–i21.

Whitley, R.J., Hayden, F.G., Reisinger, K.S., Young, N., Dutkowski, R., Ipe, D., Mills, R.G. and Ward, P. (2001) Oral oseltamivir treatment of influenza in children. *Pediatric Infectious Disease Journal* 20, 127–133.

Writing Committee of the Second World Health Organization Consultation on Clinical Aspects of Human Infection with Avian Influenza A (H5N1) Virus; Abdel-Ghafar, A.N., Chotpitayasunondh, T., Gao, Z., Hayden, F.G., Nguyen, D.H., de Jong, M.D., Naghdaliyev, A., Peiris, J.S., Shindo, N., Soeroso, S. and Uyeki, T.M. (2008) Update on avian influenza A (H5N1) virus infection in humans. *New England Journal of Medicine* 358, 261–273.

Antibiotics

British Infection Society, British Thoracic Society and Health Protection Agency (2007) Pandemic flu: clinical management of patients with an influenza-like illness during an influenza pandemic. Provisional guidelines from the British Infection Society, British Thoracic Society, and Health Protection Agency in collaboration with the Department of Health. *Thorax* 62(Suppl. 1), 1–46.

Brundage, J.F. (2006) Interactions between influenza and bacterial respiratory pathogens: implications for pandemic preparedness. *Lancet Infectious Diseases* 6, 303–312.

Brundage, J.F. and Shanks, G.D. (2008) Deaths from bacterial pneumonia during 1918–19 influenza pandemic. *Emerging Infectious Diseases* 14, 1193–1199.

Casellas, J.M., Gilardoni, M., Tome, G., Goldberg, M., Ivanovic, S., Orduna, M., Dolmann, A., Ascoli, M., Ariza, H. and Montero, J.M. (1999) Comparative *in-vitro* activity of levofloxacin against isolates of bacteria from adult patients with community-acquired lower respiratory tract infections. *Journal of Antimicrobial Chemotherapy* 43(Suppl. C), 37–42.

Gupta, R.K., George, R. and Nguyen-Van-Tam, J.S. (2008) Bacterial pneumonia and pandemic influenza planning. *Emerging Infectious Diseases* 14, 1187–1192.

McCullers, J.A. (2006) Insights into the interaction between influenza virus and pneumococcus. *Clinical Microbiology Reviews* 19, 571–582.

Morens, D.M., Taubenberger, J.K. and Fauci, A.S. (2008) Predominant role of bacterial pneumonia as a cause of death in pandemic influenza: implications for pandemic influenza preparedness. *Journal of Infectious Diseases* 198, 962–970.

Soper, G.A. (1918) The pandemic in the Army camps. *Journal of the American Medical Association* 71, 1899–1909.

Whitney, C.G., Farley, M.M., Hadler, J., Harrison, L.H., Bennett, N.M., Lynfield, R., Reingold, A., Cieslak, P.R., Pilishvili, T., Jackson, D., Facklam, R.R., Jorgensen, J.H. and Schuchat, A.; Active Bacterial Core Surveillance of the Emerging Infections Program Network (2003) Decline in invasive pneumococcal disease after the introduction of protein–polysaccharide conjugate vaccine. *New England Journal of Medicine* 348, 1737–1746.

9 Vaccines

L. HESSEL

- What will be the role of vaccination in an influenza pandemic?
- How can as much vaccine as possible be supplied as early as possible in a pandemic situation and will there be sufficient vaccines globally?
- What are the most appropriate and realistic vaccination strategies in a pandemic situation?
- How should vaccines be allocated and delivered in a pandemic situation?
- Will pandemic preparedness efforts benefit seasonal influenza vaccines and vaccination policies and, if so, in what way?

9.1 Introduction

Vaccination represents the most effective medical intervention to control influenza during epidemic (interpandemic) periods. In the event of a pandemic, a specific monovalent vaccine will have to be developed rapidly, and subsequently produced in substantial quantities. The global demand for a pandemic vaccine will result in increased pressure from health authorities, the medical community and the general public, all seeking access to the vaccine. There is, therefore, a substantial risk of inadequate, inequitable and delayed supply, including possible measures by countries with production facilities to limit or prevent export to countries without such facilities.

If an influenza pandemic occurs before adequate preparations have been made, this could result in a public health emergency of unprecedented scale and an economic crisis due to excess morbidity and mortality in adults of working age, accompanied by social disruption and panic. Hence, the need to guarantee adequate supplies of pandemic vaccine was highlighted in the resolution adopted by the 56th World Health Assembly on 28 May 2003 to ensure that all World Health Organization (WHO) Member States give priority to influenza pandemic preparedness planning. This led to the establishment by the WHO of a global pandemic influenza vaccine action plan (GAP) and development of national pandemic preparedness plans in a great many countries worldwide.

Pandemic preparedness raises many issues and challenges in terms of both vaccine availability and strategic approaches to use. The successful handling of these issues will rely upon common understanding and anticipation of the roles and responsibilities of each partner. Active collaboration between governments, public health authorities and international institutions, scientific experts and the vaccine manufacturers is needed to overcome the obstacles and to guarantee rapid access to pandemic vaccines. This collaboration includes understanding the links and differences between

©CAB International 2010. *Introduction to Pandemic Influenza*
(eds J.S. Nguyen-Van-Tam and C. Sellwood)

seasonal and pandemic vaccines, addressing the numerous challenges to develop, license, produce and distribute these vaccines, and then defining and successfully implementing appropriate vaccination strategies.

9.2   Seasonal Influenza Vaccines: the Basis for Pandemic Vaccine Development and Production

Influenza vaccine production process

Currently, the WHO recommends three different influenza viruses for inclusion in seasonal influenza vaccines: two A virus subtypes (A/H1N1 and A/H3N2) and a single B virus. As a result of the continuous genetic mutations ('drift') of influenza viruses, each year the WHO recommends which strains should be used in vaccines for the forthcoming influenza season, based on surveillance data gathered by more than 100 national influenza centres in 89 countries around the world. During the 21-year period from the 1980–1981 season to the 2001–2002 season, the vaccine composition has been changed eight times for the A/H1N1 component, 14 times for the A/H3N2 component and ten times for the influenza B component.

The influenza surveillance network and the process to prepare vaccine strains and reagents are summarized in Fig. 9.1. When a new virus strain is detected, it is sent for

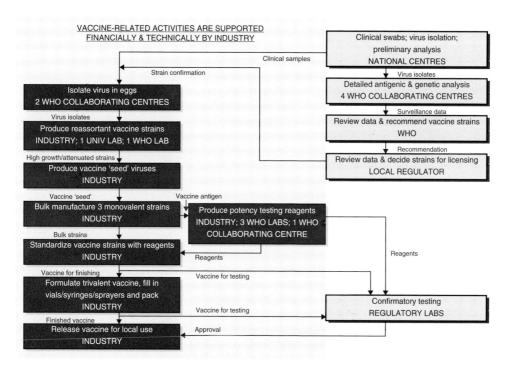

Fig. 9.1. The World Health Organization (WHO) Global Influenza Surveillance Network and preparation of standardized vaccine strains and reagents. (Courtesy of the Influenza Vaccine Supply International Task Force of the International Federation of Pharmaceutical Manufacturers & Associations.)

detailed antigenic and molecular analysis to one or more of the four WHO Collaborating Centres for Influenza Reference and Research in: London, UK; Atlanta, USA; Melbourne, Australia; and Tokyo, Japan. Twice a year, data are reviewed by the collaborating centres (in mid-February for the northern hemisphere and mid-September for the southern hemisphere) to determine which strains should be included in the following season's vaccine. This WHO recommendation is considered by the local regulatory authorities, who make the final decision on the strains to be included in vaccines for use in their territories that season.

Almost all influenza vaccines are produced by growing the virus on fertilized hens' eggs. Although seed strains for the B virus component are usually prepared from field isolates and grow well in eggs, influenza A reference viruses are not immediately suitable for manufacturing vaccines, as most wild-type A viruses do not grow efficiently in eggs. Instead, strains that are antigenically similar to the reference viruses with respect to their haemagglutinin (HA) and neuraminidase (NA) antigens, and which also possess the appropriate properties for efficient production and compliance with regulatory standards, have to be identified. The selected virus isolates are grown in hens' eggs by the WHO collaborating centres, then 'high-growth reassortant viruses' are developed by laboratories at the New York Medical College, the UK's National Institute for Biological Standards and Control (NIBSC) and the vaccine manufacturer CSL in Australia. The natural tendency of influenza viruses to reassort their genes is harnessed to create viruses containing six 'backbone' genes of a master viral strain that does grow well in eggs, such as A/Puerto Rico/8/34 (PR8), plus the two genes for the HA and NA antigens of the required vaccine strain. Once the similarity of the candidate seed strains to the reference strains has been confirmed, the candidate seed strains are sent to the vaccine manufacturers to start production. This process takes approximately 2 months.

Each of the three vaccine strains is produced separately. The working seed is injected into the allantoic cavity of embryonated hens' eggs where it multiplies rapidly. After several days of propagation, the live vaccine strain is separated from the fluid, inactivated, purified and then processed further, depending on whether the manufacturer is producing whole virus, split virus or purified surface antigen (HA and NA) vaccines (Table 9.1). Some manufacturers are beginning to deploy cell culture as an alternative method of preparing inactivated vaccines. These techniques have the theoretical advantage of removing the dependency on fertilized hens' eggs. Although not yet widely available, it is expected that these products will become more commonplace

Table 9.1. Vaccine types.

Whole	Split virion	Subunit
Whole virus grown, killed and packaged intact into the vaccine	Whole virus grown, killed, broken apart including internal proteins and packaged into the vaccine	Whole virus grown, killed, surface antigens extracted and packaged into vaccine (no internal proteins)

L. Hessel

as time progresses. Live attenuated influenza vaccines (LAIVs) are developed in a similar working seed propagation process, but do not undergo inactivation. Instead, the virus is passaged through a foreign host (e.g. tissue culture cells) to introduce mutations that will reduce virulence while maintaining immunogenicity.

To quantify the antigen content of the vaccines, the manufacturers use potency testing reagents standardized by the WHO reference laboratories. Once the antigen content has been established for each of the three strains, they are blended together to form a trivalent bulk, which is filled into vials, syringes or sprays and packed. At present, all available seasonal influenza vaccines contain 15 µg of HA for each of the three virus strains.

Each batch of vaccine must be tested to ensure it conforms to the quality standards of the local regulatory agencies. In addition, the European Medicines Evaluation Agency (EMEA) in the European Union (EU) requires that the safety and immunogenicity of each new influenza vaccine formulation is evaluated in a clinical study before the vaccine can be released for use in the EU. Similar processes exist in other parts of the world.

The vaccine production process, from issue of the WHO recommendations on the strains to be included to availability of the vaccine on the market, takes approximately 6 months (Fig. 9.2).

Production capacity

Since the mid-1990s, vaccine manufacturers have substantially increased their capability to supply influenza vaccines in response to rising demand, and this trend continues.

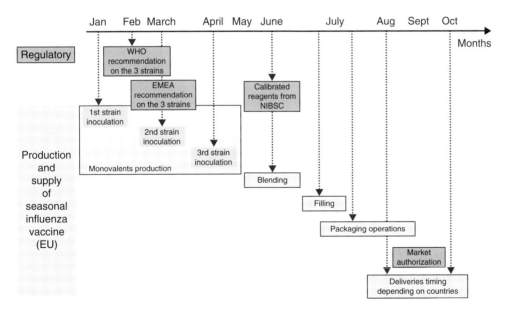

Fig. 9.2. The influenza vaccine approval and production process in the European Union (EU) (WHO, World Health Organization; EMEA, European Medicines Evaluation Agency; NIBSC, UK's National Institute for Biological Standards and Control). (Courtesy of the Influenza Vaccine Working Group of the European Vaccine Manufacturers.)

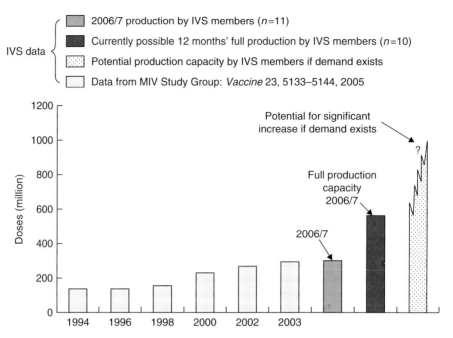

Fig. 9.3. Progress in expanding the production capacity of trivalent inactivated vaccines (IVS, Influenza Vaccine Supply International Task Force; MIV, Macro-epidemiology of Influenza Vaccination). (Courtesy of the International Federation of Pharmaceutical Manufacturers & Associations' IVS International Task Force.)

In the decade from 1994 to 2003, the number of vaccine doses distributed worldwide grew rapidly from 135 million to approximately 300 million (Fig. 9.3). A further increase, to over 408 million doses distributed worldwide, was seen by 2007. Manufacturers are continuing to invest heavily in influenza vaccine production, and anticipate more than doubling their current production capacity by 2010, pending significant increase in seasonal influenza vaccination usage.

The driver of production capacity is the uptake of vaccines. This will increase if the WHO objective of influenza vaccination coverage for at least 75% of people aged 65 years and over by 2010 is achieved. However, despite vaccination recommendations, vaccine uptake remains generally low, even in well-resourced settings. A survey of the 27 member countries of the EU plus Norway and Iceland found that coverage of people aged over 65 years during the 2006–2007 influenza season reached the WHO target of 75% only in the UK and the Netherlands. Data from Japan also show that the vaccine coverage rate for the elderly has failed to rise above approximately 50% during recent seasons, including 2006–2007. Furthermore, while vaccination is recommended for over 70% of the US population, it has been estimated that just one-third were immunized in 2006–2007.

The role of seasonal influenza vaccination in pandemic preparedness

Seasonal influenza vaccines are not expected to have a direct impact on an influenza pandemic, as the HA of the pandemic virus strain will, by definition, be antigenically

L. Hessel

distinct from that of the seasonal strains. Nevertheless, sustained use of seasonal influenza vaccines could contribute to pandemic preparedness:

- Achieving high vaccination coverage with seasonal influenza vaccines during the interpandemic period could reduce the risk of co-infection with a human and a non-human virus in the same individual, and thus reduce the likelihood of reassortment.
- Although the role of NA in the induction of immunity to influenza is not well documented, there could be some overlap between human and non-human NAs. For example, N1 could induce some level of cross-protection between A/H1N1 human strains and A/H5N1 avian viruses. Early clinical trials with A/H5N1 vaccines in the elderly have shown that a single dose of vaccine was sufficient to elicit satisfactory immune responses in elderly subjects, suggesting a 'priming' effect of earlier contacts with circulating N1 strains. However, these data are not strong enough to sustain a population-level justification not to use pandemic vaccine once it becomes available.
- In addition to the direct public health impact of increasing vaccination coverage for seasonal influenza, it will drive vaccine production, hence increasing potential production capacity for pandemic vaccines.

From seasonal to pandemic vaccines: an inextricable link

Although the final formulation of pandemic vaccines is likely to be different from seasonal vaccines (see later), their production processes are essentially the same.

Once the pandemic virus strain is identified by the WHO collaborating centres, the reassortant vaccine strain will be engineered (see later). The virus will then be provided to the vaccine manufacturers to prepare working seeds and begin bulk pandemic vaccine production. The influenza pandemic vaccines will be produced in the same manufacturing facilities as the current seasonal influenza vaccines. The reasons for this are twofold. First, the manufacturing process is inherently similar for the two types of vaccine. Second, vaccine manufacturing is a complex and lengthy process, requiring experienced and skilled employees who have specific knowledge of the production processes. All production facilities must be compliant with Good Manufacturing Practice (GMP) standards. Construction and formal validation of a new facility takes up to 5 years; consequently, any vaccine production plant therefore requires not only a significant initial investment, but also major ongoing investment to maintain GMP conditions, quality and regulatory standards and to ensure sustainability. For a production plant to remain GMP-compliant, retain the necessary highly-qualified staff and be ready to produce pandemic influenza vaccines, it must be used regularly. It is neither practical nor realistic to have idle manufacturing capacity that could be 'switched on' during a pandemic. Even for a state-owned facility where such a decision could be made if appropriately skilled staff and the necessary resources and equipment were readily available, such a strategy would be highly questionable in terms of the return on investment. The optimal use of such plants is, therefore, for the production of seasonal influenza vaccines. Thus, investing in manufacturing capacity for seasonal vaccines should be seen as inextricably linked to overall pandemic preparedness.

9.3 The Key Challenges of Pandemic Vaccine Development and Production

Research and development

Identifying novel viruses with pandemic potential is critical to ensure early development of a pandemic vaccine. Since the late 1990s, several strains of avian influenza virus have caused disease in man, including A/H5N1, at least three A/H7 subtypes and A/H9N2, and all of these have pandemic potential. In addition, the process of antigenic recycling (see Chapter 2) would suggest that an A/H2 virus is another potential pandemic precursor. Nevertheless, as a result of its unprecedented panzootic impact and its sporadic transmission to people over the past decade, the A/H5N1 subtype is the focus of much of the current research and development (R&D) activities.

Irrespective of the virus type, one of the challenges in the development of avian influenza vaccines has been to generate suitable virus strains that can be grown in eggs, as viruses such as A/H5N1 and A/H7N7, which are highly pathogenic in poultry, kill fertilized hens' eggs as well as live birds. This has been achieved using 'reverse genetics' to construct the vaccine seed. First, the genes coding for HA and NA from the A/H5N1 strain are modified to render them non-virulent. Then, as in the preparation of seasonal vaccine viruses, the modified HA and NA genes are combined with six genes from a virus that can grow in eggs. Reverse genetics can be used to generate all types of vaccine (live, inactivated and subunit vaccines).

Another challenge for the development of pandemic vaccines is the availability of immunological tools and animal models to assess their potential efficacy. Although animal challenge studies, especially in ferrets, can provide useful data on vaccine efficacy against homologous and heterologous (drift variants) to the vaccine virus, they cannot be routinely used. Antigen-specific, anti-HA antibody titres, measured in the haemagglutination-inhibition assay, are generally accepted as a marker of efficacy for influenza vaccines, and are used for the registration of the seasonal influenza vaccines. However, although they are an official legal and regulatory standard for licensure, such methods are not strongly correlated to clinical efficacy and are not necessarily relevant to measure the immunogenicity of pandemic vaccines. Indeed, with regard to pandemic vaccines, this correlate is heavily questioned by most experts. Other potential correlates of immunity against influenza need to be investigated, for example antibodies against NA and M2 protein and markers of cell-mediated responses. Their use and value in the assessment of immune responses to vaccination are being investigated through collaborative studies to establish international standards.

Another challenge is to maximize the number of vaccine doses that can be produced, by using the lowest concentration of antigen necessary to induce a protective immune response. Several approaches are being investigated and are summarized in following sections.

As it is never possible to predict when pandemics will emerge, vaccine manufacturers are looking at both short- and medium- to long-term approaches to the development of pandemic vaccines. The short-term approach relies upon the application of existing technology, knowledge and manufacturing facilities for seasonal influenza vaccines to produce prototype pandemic vaccines using avian strains with pandemic potential. Such vaccines are used in clinical trials designed to define the optimal formulation for the actual pandemic vaccine. By December 2008, nine

L. Hessel

Library and eLearning Centre
Gartnavel General Hospital

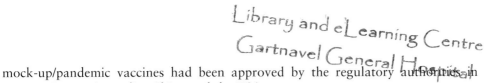

mock-up/pandemic vaccines had been approved by the regulatory authorities in Europe, Japan, Australia, China and the USA.

The medium- to long-term approach focuses on improving vaccine performance, including the development of new vaccines that allow antigen-sparing, broad-spectrum and long-lasting immunity, other production technologies, alternative antigen delivery systems, and new vaccine concepts (see later). The ultimate goal is the development of a 'universal' influenza vaccine that protects against any influenza strain. The potential of influenza vaccines that can elicit protective antibodies against highly conserved viral proteins (e.g. M2) is therefore also being investigated.

These R&D activities require considerable investment by the vaccine manufacturers to develop vaccines that might not be used. By the end of 2008, industry had voluntarily invested over US$4 billion to protect society against pandemic influenza.

Regulatory issues

As with all vaccines, pandemic influenza vaccines will need to be licensed by the appropriate local regulatory authorities. To expedite the licensing process and availability of pandemic influenza vaccines, specific registration processes have been developed based on the concept of 'mock-up' vaccines.

A mock-up pandemic influenza vaccine can contain any influenza virus subtype to which man has not yet been widely exposed, such as A/H5N1, A/H5N3, A/H7N7 and A/H9N2. In all other respects, the vaccine composition and manufacturing methods are those that will be used for the pandemic influenza vaccine. The necessary pre-clinical tests and clinical trials of immunogenicity and safety are carried out with the mock-up vaccine, to predict how people will react to vaccination with the pandemic virus strain. The mock-up dossier should also include a plan to monitor the vaccine's efficacy and safety after registration (a risk management plan). Once the regulators are satisfied that all the necessary criteria have been met, the mock-up vaccine is granted a licence, although it is a condition of licensure that the product is not used. This is simply a clever manoeuvre, so that once a pandemic is declared, the manufacturer will produce the vaccine according to the formulation and process validated with the mock-up, but using the real pandemic influenza virus strain. As the rest of the relevant data will already have been reviewed during assessment of the mock-up vaccine, the registration process will consist of a variation to the vaccine's marketing authorization limited to the characteristics of the new strain. Therefore, it is anticipated that by this route the marketing authorization of the pandemic vaccine will be shortened from 12 months or more to 1–2 weeks. This innovative regulatory process is of considerable public health importance because it will greatly speed up the time it takes to licence a pandemic vaccine in an emergency. However, only those manufacturers with a mock-up vaccine licensed in advance will be able to utilize this procedure.

Under normal circumstances, the vaccine manufacturers/marketing authorization holders are responsible for any liabilities arising from the use of their vaccines. However, exposure to pandemic influenza vaccines will differ from that for regular marketed vaccines. The final vaccine is likely to have different characteristics from the strain used for registration (i.e. the mock-up vaccine), it will be used before complete clinical data have been obtained, and it will be administered through mass vaccination campaigns conducted by governments. Risk management plans therefore need to be defined with the relevant health authorities and provision made to temporarily waive or limit the liability of manufacturers with regard to vaccine adverse experiences. Specific liability measures have been agreed between the vaccine manufacturers and the relevant authorities in Australia, the USA and some European countries.

Manufacturing aspects

Pandemic vaccines will differ from seasonal influenza vaccines in several ways that will influence production capacity. First, the pandemic vaccines will be monovalent instead of trivalent, which suggests that the production capacity for the pandemic vaccine can be three times higher than for a seasonal vaccine. In addition, whole virus vaccines that increase the supply of antigen compared with the split virus or subunit vaccines for seasonal influenza, or the use of an adjuvant to allow reduced antigen content per dose compared with seasonal vaccines, will increase the number of doses produced each week. Conversely, if the production yield of the pandemic virus strain is inferior to that of seasonal influenza strains, the number of doses that can be produced will also be lower.

9.4   Current Status of Pandemic Vaccine Development and Future Prospects

Development of avian influenza vaccines

A wide range of research concepts for new influenza vaccines has been explored to develop potential vaccines against avian strains with pandemic potential, including: inactivated whole cell, split or subunit vaccines; live attenuated virus vaccines; the use of adjuvants and other immune-enhancing mechanisms (e.g. virosomes); other production technologies (cell culture, vector expression); alternative antigen delivery systems (intranasal, intradermal, transcutaneous); and new vaccine concepts (DNA vaccines and M2 antigens) (Table 9.2).

Each of these approaches has both advantages and disadvantages. For example, cell-culture techniques can increase manufacturing flexibility and robustness, be scaled up to meet increased demand for vaccine, and safeguard against any possible production risk related to a lethal effect of avian influenza viruses on hens' eggs. However, it has other regulatory constraints and there is very limited experience of

Table 9.2. Progress in pandemic vaccine development.

Vaccine types	Production methods	Adjuvants	Delivery systems	Novel vaccine concepts
Inactivated: whole virus split virus subunit	Embryonated hens' eggs Cell culture: MDCK Vero	Aluminium salts MF59 AS03 AF03	Injection: intramuscular subcutaneous Intradermal	DNA vaccines M2 vaccines
Live attenuated virus	PER.C6		Intranasal	

L. Hessel

using this process for producing seasonal influenza vaccines at the present time. Therefore, egg-based production currently remains the universal standard against which other production methods are judged, and is likely to remain the main source for most pandemic vaccines in the short to medium term.

Similarly, inactivated whole-cell vaccines and LAIVs have potential advantages compared with split virion and subunit vaccines, including greater immunogenicity and cross-protection against other influenza virus strains. In addition, LAIVs are administered intranasally, which provides the opportunity to induce antibodies at the mucosa of the respiratory tract. However, as LAIVs retain the ability to replicate, they could mutate to a new pathogenic strain.

Measures to enhance the immunogenicity of inactivated vaccines with the addition of adjuvants or alternative delivery routes could be associated with an increased risk of adverse reactions.

Finally, the efficacy of novel vaccine concepts (such as DNA and M2 vaccines) has not been established.

Although the majority of vaccines studied in clinical trials so far have been directed against the A/H5N1 strain, vaccines directed against other strains, including A/H5N3, A/H7N3, A/H7N7 and A/H9N2, have also been investigated. As part of pandemic preparedness planning, libraries of candidate viruses for vaccine production would be of great value.

Antigen sparing

As most people will be immunologically naive to the pandemic strain, it is anticipated that two doses of the pandemic vaccine will be required to provide full protection, impacting de facto on the number of doses needed. The ability to use the lowest possible dose of vaccine to promote a protective immune response will, therefore, optimize vaccine supply and maximize global public health benefit. This was deemed especially necessary as high antigen content, of up to $90\,\mu$g HA per dose, was found to be necessary to elicit immune responses to the first A/H5N1 candidate vaccine.

Addition of an adjuvant to the vaccine formulation can enhance the immune response to vaccination, thereby improving efficacy and potentially reducing the amount of antigen per dose. This potential antigen sparing could substantially increase the number of pandemic influenza vaccine doses available (Fig. 9.4). For example, the opportunity to vaccinate using $2\times3.8\,\mu$g doses of vaccine instead of $2\times15\,\mu$g doses would quadruple the number of people who could be immunized.

Potential adjuvant candidates include aluminium salts and the oil-in-water emulsions MF59 (Novartis), AS03 (GlaxoSmithKline) and AF03 (Sanofi Pasteur). While studies with A/H5N1 vaccines that used aluminium hydroxide as an adjuvant have shown only limited benefits for the immunogenicity of split virion and whole-cell vaccines, enhanced immunogenicity has been reported for vaccines that included oil-in-water adjuvants. Although adjuvanted vaccines tend to induce more local and systemic reactions than plain formulations and further clinical studies of their efficacy are needed, the prospect for antigen sparing appears to be realistic.

Notwithstanding, one manufacturer (Baxter) has successfully developed a wild-type A/H5N1 vaccine based on cell culture, which does not require adjuvant yet has similar antigen-sparing characteristics.

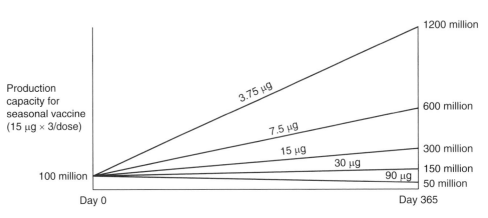

*Assuming same yield for pandemic vaccine as for seasonal strains

Fig. 9.4. The impact of antigen sparing on pandemic vaccine production. (Courtesy of the European Vaccine Manufacturers' Influenza Working Group.)

Cross-protection between clades: the basis for 'pre-pandemic' vaccination

Antigenic drift is a feature of influenza viruses, including highly pathogenic avian strains. It is therefore important that a pandemic vaccine can provide protection against not only the specific strain with which it was prepared, but also any variants ('clades') that may subsequently emerge. If this can be achieved, it might also be possible to consider using vaccines made from the avian virus precursor of the pandemic strain adapted to direct human-to-human transmission as a first line of defence when the pandemic is declared, until the first pandemic vaccine batches are available.

Clinical studies with A/H5N1 vaccine candidates have found evidence that they can provide cross-protection against different mutant clades of the same avian strain. For example, a clade 1 A/H5N1 vaccine provided cross-protection against A/H5N1 subclades 2.1, 2.2 and 2.3, while an A/H5N3 vaccine with MF59 provided cross-protection against A/H5N1. In addition, studies in a mouse model with LAIVs grown in a continuous cell culture system have shown that a clade 1 A/H5N1 vaccine provided protection against the homologous strain and also against a clade 2 strain, and vice versa.

Thus, the ability to induce cross-protection between clades gives the potential for so-called 'pre-pandemic' vaccination strategies. This concept relies on the use of vaccines from avian influenza strains with pandemic potential to provide protection in the early stage of the pandemic before the actual pandemic strain, derived from the same avian strain, is fully characterized and the corresponding vaccine is developed. It also offers the possibility of stockpiling such vaccines so that they would be immediately available at the start of the pandemic, or could be given in advance. Some governments have already procured stockpiles of human A/H5N1 vaccine for these purposes.

The concept of 'pre-pandemic' vaccine nevertheless needs to be tempered with a certain degree of understanding of the potential risks. It is quite impossible to predict the subtype of the next human pandemic, although there is no question that A/H5N1

L. Hessel

presents a major risk. However, a vaccine against A/H5N1 would not be expected to have any protective affect against an A/H7 or A/H9 virus, for example. Thus the term 'pre-pandemic', while well established, would be a misnomer. There is an inherent risk associated with being unable to predict the next pandemic virus subtype and this risk in relation to pre-pandemic vaccine will remain until a multivalent product with antigens targeted against the 'top-four' pandemic threats (A/H2, A/H5, A/H7 and A/H9) is developed.

9.5 Vaccination Policies and Pandemic Preparedness

Objectives and expected impact

Vaccination strategies and priorities depend on the objectives. The overall goal of vaccination is to minimize the impact of an influenza pandemic by protecting individuals and the community against the infection. By reducing the morbidity and mortality associated with pandemic influenza, social disruption and the economic consequences of increased demand for medical services, healthcare costs and lost productivity will be limited.

As the pandemic vaccines will be available only progressively at the outset of the pandemic (i.e. in small quantities at first until production scales up), each government will have to plan in advance and determine the priority groups for vaccination. Some governments have already placed advance orders with manufacturers, in order to secure a priority position for early delivery. Ideally, if sufficient supply is available the entire population should be vaccinated with the pandemic vaccine. However, if vaccine supply is limited, healthcare workers and other key workers required to maintain the country's critical infrastructure should be vaccinated as a priority. Interestingly, modelling has shown that a staged vaccination programme has maximum effect on reducing transmission if children are vaccinated first, since school-aged children have the highest transmission rates. Vaccinating children first might also be ethically and morally acceptable to the general public.

Vaccination strategies: pandemic versus pre-pandemic vaccination and the role of mathematical modelling

One major drawback of vaccination strategies during a pandemic is that, according to the current influenza vaccine production timelines, it will take 3–6 months from the pandemic declaration until the first supplies of pandemic vaccine are available. Consequently, a pandemic influenza vaccine will not be available in time to prevent the first wave of infection, although it will be able to prevent or ameliorate subsequent waves if they occur. In this context it should also be stressed that a pandemic virus in effect becomes the 'normal' seasonal influenza virus after the pandemic has passed. For example, after the A/H3N2 pandemic in 1968, the virus did not disappear, but instead became the dominant seasonal virus which persists until the present day (Chapter 1). After a pandemic, the first few winter seasonal epidemics are often severe. Thus a pandemic vaccine that misses the first pandemic wave still offers considerable public health benefit. To address this delay, several authorities, including the WHO, are considering the potential for the 'pre-pandemic' vaccination concept, which could be implemented from WHO Pandemic Alert Phase 4. This approach relies upon the ability of vaccines prepared against one or more of the avian influenza strains genetically related to the predicted pandemic virus to provide cross-protection against the actual pandemic strain, as has been shown for A/H5N1 vaccines (see above).

Different strategies for the use of pre-pandemic vaccines are being considered (Fig. 9.5):

- Using a stockpile of pre-pandemic vaccines in selected populations immediately at the start of the pandemic, to be followed with a dose of pandemic vaccine when this becomes available.
- Using a monovalent pre-pandemic vaccine for priming during the interpandemic period, followed by a booster dose of the pandemic vaccine after onset of the pandemic. A larger proportion of the population could then be immunized more quickly against the pandemic strain than with the stockpile approach.
- Using stand-alone vaccination programmes, comprising two doses of pre-pandemic vaccine given in advance of a pandemic, would spread the vaccination programme across many years, rather than requiring a surge in vaccine production when a pandemic is declared. It could also provide a long-term approach towards immunization against several potential pandemic strains.

The feasibility of such strategies is subject to several constraints. Vaccines intended for pre-pandemic use must undergo the regular licensing procedure for vaccines, including a more extensive pre-licensure clinical development, defined by precise guidelines in Europe, rather than the more limited process for mock-up pandemic vaccines described earlier. By October 2008, the EMEA had licensed one A/H5N1 vaccine for pre-pandemic use vaccine for use in Europe, and pre-pandemic vaccines had also been licensed in China and Japan.

Beyond these regulatory aspects, several issues must be addressed, including the selection of the virus clade, the actual clinical efficacy of these vaccines, the political

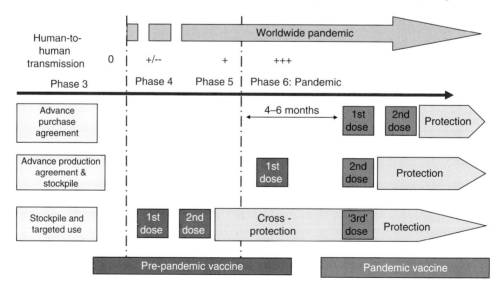

Fig. 9.5. Potential vaccination strategies for pandemic influenza. (Courtesy of the European Vaccine Manufacturers' Influenza Working Group.)

L. Hessel

and ethical decision to immunize individuals against a non-human disease, prioritization of target populations, safety aspects and subsequent potential liability. Despite these issues, and the unknown clinical efficacy of pre-pandemic vaccines, the WHO and healthcare policy makers in several countries have recognized the potential value of this approach and are establishing stockpiles of human vaccines against avian A/H5N1.

Indeed, despite the expectation of a lower efficacy compared with the actual pandemic vaccines, evidence from mathematical modelling studies has provided support for the pre-pandemic vaccinations strategies to limit the impact of a pandemic.

Focus Box 9.1. Mathematical modelling and vaccination strategies to address the pandemic threat.

In the absence of evidence from clinical studies regarding the effectiveness of vaccination against pandemic influenza, mathematical modelling is an invaluable tool to assess the potential impact of vaccination strategies to control a pandemic situation, alone or in combination with other medical and non-medical countermeasures.

Although few in number, sophisticated models have been developed and provide useful tools to manage this complex policy-making process. First, the models showed that combination strategies are needed, and that the timing of their implementation is critical for success. Second, rapid deployment is a key goal, as delaying the transmission of the virus by non-medical intervention will translate into days or weeks of vaccine production. Third, assuming minimum cross-protection between the avian strain related to the pandemic virus, modelling supports pre-pandemic vaccination by reducing the number of susceptible individuals first exposed to the pandemic virus, especially if a first dose provides some degree of protection or if it can prime the immune system so that only one dose of the pandemic vaccine is needed.

A stochastic influenza simulation model suggests that the rapid production and distribution of pre-pandemic vaccines, even if poorly matched to the pandemic strain, could significantly slow the spread of disease and limit the number of people affected. For example, assuming a reproduction number $R_0=2$, vaccinating all the population with a vaccine that has an efficacy of as little as 20% would reduce an overall attack rate of about 35% without vaccine to 20%. The effect is particularly important when combined with other countermeasures such as antivirals. Combined with antiviral treatment, school closures and antiviral prophylaxis of household contacts, even limited (i.e. less than 50%) coverage of a such a pre-pandemic vaccine could bring the reproduction number down to less than the self-sustaining threshold, $R_0=1$. In this case there would be no national epidemic of pandemic influenza and only a limited number of local outbreaks.

Finally, models suggest that vaccination programmes produce the greatest reductions in transmission if children are vaccinated first, as school-aged children have the highest transmission rates.

Nevertheless, even if mathematical modelling supports pre-pandemic vaccination, strategic issues still need to be addressed regarding the size of a stockpile, the time to acquire it versus the risk of antigenic drift between the avian and human pandemic strains, and the possibility of producing large amounts of pre-pandemic vaccines and using them before the pandemic vaccine is available. Managing uncertainty is the key challenge in pandemic preparedness.

Operational issues: allocation, distribution and stockpiling of vaccines

In addition to the work performed by the vaccine manufacturers to develop and produce pandemic influenza vaccines, governments need to finalize their vaccination strategies and establish reasonable forecasts for vaccine requirements, which can form the basis for contractual agreements with manufacturers for the procurement of (pre-pandemic and) pandemic vaccines.

Governments and international organizations also need to define equitable vaccine allocation and procurement processes for all countries. This includes developing the necessary infrastructure for vaccine distribution and delivery, and/or strengthening existing systems, to meet the demand for rapid vaccination.

The process for shipping pandemic vaccine from the manufacturer to inventory centres and subsequent distribution to vaccinators must be planned. Appropriate communication lines also need to be established in advance of a pandemic. Public health systems must be able to collect, stock, distribute and deliver vaccines to the targeted population. Most pandemic vaccines will probably be formulated with an adjuvant (with mixing of the two components in the syringe immediately prior to injection) and two doses will be required to provide full protection. The logistics of managing the vaccination process therefore need to be planned. The stockpiling and distribution of syringes and needles also need to be included in planning for a pandemic vaccination programme. The vaccine will need to be stored in approved warehouses and, together with the supply chain, will require appropriate security. Sadly, plans also need to be made to deal with the inevitable counterfeit vaccines that will appear.

Many of the same considerations apply when establishing and maintaining stockpiles of pre-pandemic vaccines. In addition, the facilities in which they are stored will have to allow for the maintenance and update of stock over time, possibly at different intervals according to the shelf-life of the vaccines and adjuvants.

Complementary vaccination strategies (pneumococcal vaccines)

Historically, bacterial superinfections have been the major cause of death during past influenza pandemics, with *Streptococcus pneumoniae* the dominant pathogen. The ability to provide appropriate intensive care and broad-spectrum antibiotics to manage these infections will be compromised if clinical attack rates approach 25–30%, as seen in previous pandemics. Pandemic planning must therefore take into account the fact that bacterial pneumonia will be a frequent complication in at least 10–15% of people who survive the primary pandemic influenza infection. As already recognized by some countries, pandemic preparedness plans should therefore include pneumococcal vaccine strategies and stockpiles.

9.6 The Impact of Pandemic Influenza on Seasonal Influenza Vaccines

The interrelationship between seasonal and pandemic influenza vaccines is evident. This means that activities directed towards development of pandemic vaccines will also benefit the seasonal vaccines, including progress in R&D, production and policies.

L. Hessel

Approaches in R&D described in this chapter and new methods for assessing the immunogenicity and efficacy of influenza vaccines can be applied to improve the efficacy of seasonal vaccines.

Investment by the vaccine manufacturers in production facilities to meet the anticipated demand for pandemic vaccines has also resulted in increased production capacity for seasonal influenza vaccines. New production technology will also contribute to enhance the manufacturers' ability to scale up production in response to increasing demand.

As far as policies are concerned, it is anticipated that governments will aim to increase vaccine coverage for seasonal influenza to encourage the manufacturers to increase capacity. This could require changes to national vaccination recommendations and strategies, especially if the WHO targets are to be achieved. This will provide direct public health benefits for the control of seasonal epidemics. Similarly, consideration of the logistics of distribution and optimal delivery of pandemic influenza vaccines could help to improve annual vaccination campaigns.

Taken together, the various aspects of pandemic preparedness planning in relation to vaccines can be expected to improve the development and usage of seasonal influenza vaccines.

9.7 Conclusion

To conclude, an influenza pandemic poses a major threat, not only for the general population and public health authorities, but also for the vaccine industry in terms of R&D, marketing authorization and production capacity. The successful handling of these issues will rely upon common understanding of the roles and responsibilities of each partner. Anticipation and active collaboration between governments, international organizations, industry and academia is needed to overcome the obstacles and to guarantee the most rapid development, production and use of vaccines. Significant progress has been made in pandemic preparedness since the beginning of the 21st century, including sustained industry efforts at both R&D and production levels. Key elements have also been identified that should be addressed to ensure timely and equitable access of vaccines to the population in case of an influenza pandemic. But, unless political, healthcare and financial landscapes evolve rapidly from their present status, many countries in resource-poor situations will encounter extreme difficulties in securing timely, population-wide access to pandemic vaccines when available, despite the considerable efforts of the WHO, the United Nations and the international community.

9.8 Summary Points

- In combination with other medical and non-medical countermeasures, vaccination may prove the most important strategy in containing or controlling an influenza pandemic, both by reducing the severity of disease in people who are infected and the transmission of the pandemic strain, provided appropriate approaches are anticipated and developed.
- Rapid progress in R&D could potentially solve the pandemic supply issue and make pre-pandemic strategies a reality, especially through antigen sparing, adjuvant

technology and production capacity, assuming continued growth in seasonal vaccine usage. Use of a pre-pandemic vaccine to prime immunity followed by a 'booster' of specific pandemic vaccine is an effective way to immunize as many people as possible as quickly as possible. Nevertheless, pre-pandemic vaccination carries an unavoidable risk related to the unknown identity of the next pandemic virus.

- Understanding the various factors that impact influenza vaccine manufacturing processes and capacities is essential for the formulation of policies to protect society against the significant threat of seasonal and pandemic influenza.

- Scientific advancement now justifies an emphasis on effective implementation: governments and international organizations must identify their pandemic vaccine requirements, define their pre- and pandemic vaccination strategies, plan their allocation and procurement processes with manufacturers, and ensure that critical health systems and infrastructure are in place for rapid distribution and delivery of the vaccine.

- In many respects, pandemic preparedness is inextricably linked to seasonal influenza vaccination: (i) whether for seasonal, pre-pandemic or pandemic use, influenza vaccines are manufactured in the same facilities utilizing similar processes; and (ii) improvements in R&D, and production of pandemic influenza vaccines should lead to improved seasonal influenza vaccines and long-term control of this complex disease. The sustainability of pandemic influenza vaccine supply is dependent upon seasonal usage. Increasing seasonal flu vaccine use protects society and increases pandemic capacity. As seasonal vaccine usage drives the demand for production capacity, increasing vaccination levels also boosts manufacturers' capacities to produce pandemic vaccines.

Acknowledgements

As a current member and former chairman of two working groups dedicated to influenza pandemic preparedness, the author wishes to acknowledge the major contributions of the Influenza Vaccine Supply (IVS) International Task Force of the International Federation of Pharmaceutical Manufacturers & Associations (IFPMA), and of the Influenza Vaccine Working Group of the European Vaccine Manufacturers (EVM), to the content of this chapter and the achievements described therein.

Further Reading

Ehrlich, H.J., Müller, M., Oh, H.M., Tambyah, P.A., Joukhadar, C., Montomoli, E., Fisher, D., Berezuk, G., Fritsch, S., Löw-Baselli, A., Vartian, N., Bobrovsky, R., Pavlova, B.G., Pöllabauer, E.M., Kistner, O. and Barrett, P.N.; Baxter H5N1 Pandemic Influenza Vaccine Clinical Study Team (2008) A clinical trial of a whole-virus H5N1 vaccine derived from cell culture. *New England Journal of Medicine* 358, 2573–2584.

El Sahly, H.M. and Keitel, W.A. (2000) Pandemic H5N1 influenza vaccine development: an update. *Expert Review of Vaccines* 7, 241–247.

European Centre for Disease Prevention and Control (2007) *Technical Report of the Expert Advisory Groups on Human H5N1 Vaccines: Public Health and Operational Questions,*

Stockholm, August 2007. http://ecdc.europa.eu/pdf/PH%20Questions%20final.pdf (accessed May 2009).

European Centre for Disease Prevention and Control (2007) *Technical Report of the Expert Advisory Groups on Human H5N1 Vaccines: Scientific Questions, Stockholm, August 2007.* http://ecdc.europa.eu/pdf/Sci%20Questions%20final.pdf (accessed May 2009).

European Vaccine Manufacturers (2009) Homepage. http://www.evm-vaccines.org/#/influenza/ (accessed May 2009).

Ferguson, N., Cummings, D.A., Fraser, C., Cajka, J.C., Cooley, P.C. and Burke, D.S. (2006) Strategies for mitigating an influenza pandemic. *Nature* 442, 448–452.

Gerdil, C. (2003) The annual production cycle for influenza vaccine. *Vaccine* 21, 1776–1779.

Hehme, N., Colegate, T., Palache, B. and Hessel, L. (2008) Influenza vaccine supply: building long-term sustainability. *Vaccine* 26S, D23–D26.

International Federation of Pharmaceutical Manufacturers & Associations (2009) Influenza Vaccine Supply International Task Force homepage. http://www.ifpma.org/Influenza/index.aspx (accessed May 2009).

Leroux-Roels, I., Borkowski, A., Vanwolleghem, T., Dramé, M., Clement, F., Devaster, J.M. and Leroux-Roels, G. (2007) Antigen sparing and cross-reactive immunity with an adjuvanted rH5N1 prototype pandemic influenza vaccine: a randomised controlled trial *Lancet* 370, 580–589.

World Health Organization (2006) Global pandemic influenza action plan to increase vaccine supply. http://www.who.int/csr/resources/publications/influenza/CDS_EPR_GIP_2006_1.pdf (accessed May 2009).

10 National and International Public Health Countermeasures

A. NICOLL AND H. NEEDHAM

- What is meant by the term public health countermeasures?
- From the available data and analyses, what could be the value of public health countermeasures in terms of health outcomes?
- What are the potential costs, secondary effects, risks and practical experience of the suggested countermeasures?
- Can the same countermeasures be applied in all circumstances?
- What suggested measures are likely to be the most helpful and which the least?

10.1 Introduction

In the context of seasonal and pandemic influenza, public health countermeasures can be defined as group actions taken that are intended to reduce human-to-human transmission of influenza and by that way mitigate the adverse effects of an epidemic or pandemic. Some actions are really individual actions designed to give personal protection (e.g. hand washing, mask wearing) or even treatment (e.g. taking of antiviral drugs and use of vaccines), but when taken en masse can result in overall reductions in transmission and so have a public health benefit.

The most effective countermeasure will be a specific pandemic vaccine available for the whole population. However, vaccines that match the pandemic strain of influenza are not likely to be developed, produced, licensed, available and distributed in any quantity until some months after the pandemic begins. These specific vaccines are unlikely to be available for the first wave of a pandemic strain (see Chapter 9). It is possible, if not likely, that both antiviral drugs and vaccines targeted at pandemic influenza will not be available in many parts of the world, especially in resource-poor settings. Thus, non-pharmaceutical public health countermeasures will potentially be of importance in many settings as the only effective interventions available.

10.2 Rationale and Objectives

The application of public health countermeasures is aimed at reducing the number of people who are infected, need medical care and die during an influenza pandemic. By lowering the peak of a pandemic curve and reducing the numbers affected (Fig. 10.1), the measures can also lessen the secondary consequences of pandemics that will result when many people fall sick at the same time, such as the impact of mass absenteeism on key functions (e.g. delivering healthcare, food supplies, fuel distribution,

©CAB International 2010. *Introduction to Pandemic Influenza*
(eds J.S. Nguyen-Van-Tam and C. Sellwood)

Prime objective
• Reduce transmission and so number of infections, illness and deaths
Secondary objectives
• Delay and flatten outbreak peak
• Reduce peak burden on healthcare system
• Buy some time for preparation, and developing pandemic vaccines

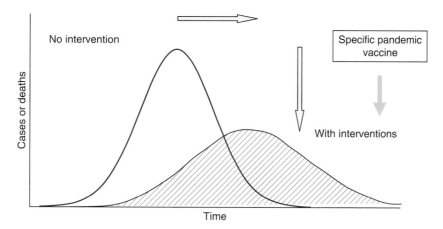

Fig. 10.1. Objectives of applying public health measures in a pandemic.

utilities, etc.). They may even push back the epidemic curve of a pandemic to a point where influenza transmission declines naturally in the summer months, or when a pandemic vaccine starts to become more widely available. This chapter focuses on measures that would be taken during World Health Organization (WHO) Pandemic Alert Phases 5 and 6 of a pandemic. It does not address the somewhat different circumstances of Phase 4 and especially the unique needs of the first emergence of a putative pandemic strain, nor the complex planning and policy issues that arise over how to sustain key services in a pandemic (i.e. business continuity planning; see Chapter 6).

A range of interventions have been suggested as public health countermeasures (Table 10.1), including personal actions enacted on a population basis (e.g. hand washing and mask wearing) and pharmaceutical interventions (e.g. antivirals and influenza vaccines). Some are simple actions to be taken by large numbers of individuals (e.g. regular hand washing and early self-isolation), while others require preparation by communities (e.g. closing schools/dismissing classes and cancelling large meetings). For many years non-pharmaceutical public health countermeasures were the only options. Nevertheless, their use varied between countries during the three pandemics of the 20th century with the greatest uptake in North America. This chapter aims to summarize what can be said about their likely effectiveness, costs (direct and indirect), their acceptability, public expectations and other more practical considerations. A more detailed appraisal of personal measures appears in Chapter 5, and of antiviral drugs, antibiotics and vaccines in Chapters 8 and 9.

It is thought that combinations of measures will be even more effective than single measures, so-called 'defence in depth' or 'layered interventions'. This is probably the case but it has to be remembered that no measures are cost-free (see below) and

Table 10.1. Public health measures for reducing influenza transmission.

Travel measures – restrictions on international travel	1. Travel advice
	2. Entry screening
	3. Border closures or severe travel restrictions
Personal protective measures	4. Regular hand washing
	5. Good respiratory hygiene (use and disposal of tissues)
	6. General mask wearing outside the home
	7. Mask wearing in high-risk public settings (non-health)
	8. Mask wearing by people with respiratory infections
	9. Early self-isolation of ill people
	10. Quarantine measures
Social distancing measures[a]	11. Internal travel restrictions
	12. Reactive school closures
	13. Proactive school closures
	14. Reactive workplace closures
	15. Home working and reducing meetings
	16. Cancelling public gatherings, international events, etc.
Antivirals – early treatment	17. All those with symptoms
	18. Health and social care and/or 'essential' workers
Antivirals – prophylaxis following a case	19. Family
	20. Family and other social contacts
	21. Family and geographical contacts
Antivirals – continuous prophylaxis	22. Health and social care and/or 'essential' workers
Vaccines – human–animal influenza vaccine ('pre-pandemic' vaccine)	23. Whole population
	24. Health and social care and/or 'essential' workers
	25. Children first
Vaccines – specific pandemic vaccine	26. Pandemic-specific vaccines

Measures are listed in no particular order of preference or hierarchy.
[a]Note that most authorities recommend using the term 'social distancing' sparingly and not grouping together individual measures. Rather, each should be considered on its own merits.

that attractive as combining measures may be to increase protection, this will inevitably increase their overall cost. A few of the measures are relatively straightforward to implement (e.g. hand washing) while others will be difficult to execute (e.g. timely mass use of antivirals by those becoming sick), and yet others are costly and potentially highly disruptive (e.g. border closures).

10.3 Effectiveness and Secondary Effects

The effectiveness of most of the measures cannot be readily predicted and a number are controversial. Effectiveness is likely to vary according to the characteristics of any pandemic so that it will *not* be possible to have set plans for either every pandemic

A. Nicoll and H. Needham

or all countries and settings. However, there will need to be default plans (plans that will be implemented in the absence of other information), which should be applied with considerable flexibility and preferably within command and control structures that will allow rapid changes to be made. There are more gaps than knowledge concerning the effectiveness and secondary effects of most measures and many will require careful consideration. The more drastic societal measures that have been suggested (e.g. proactive school closures and travel restrictions) have significant costs and consequences that will themselves vary according to setting. What experience there is with these disruptive measures shows that they are difficult to sustain. Hence for ordinary seasonal influenza or a mild, or even moderate pandemic, their application, and especially their early application, could be more damaging than just allowing the infection to run its course and treating those with more severe illness.

10.4 Timing and Implementation

Early assessment of the strategic parameters of an evolving pandemic will be crucial in deciding what public health measures should be applied. Some like the easier personal measures (e.g. routine hand washing and early self-isolation when becoming ill) should be applied under all circumstances. There is benefit in countries rehearsing their policy options for these measures, guided by the recommendations of WHO and the guidance issued by bodies like the European Centre for Disease Prevention and Control. Because of the diversity of countries, a 'one size fits all' approach will not be appropriate. However, common discussions on the measures will be helpful and more efficient and some countries have already undertaken considerable amounts of relevant scientific work, some of which this chapter draws upon.

Even within a comprehensive book such as this it is not possible to go through the relevant parameters individually for each measure, namely:

- the objective and rationale;
- the evidence of effectiveness or what is considered to be the likely effectiveness and benefits;
- the direct costs of the measure;
- the secondary effects such as indirect costs, risks and potential adverse effects;
- the likely acceptability and expectations in Europe;
- practicalities, experience and other issues; and
- WHO policy recommendations.

Instead, each one is summarized in Table 10.2.

10.5 The Measures

Scientific evidence and experience

The scientific evidence on the effectiveness of the measures generally contains more gaps than certainty. To an extent this reflects significant large gaps in knowledge about the basic characteristics of influenza transmission (see Chapter 5). There have been examinations of existing data and historical information on the measures

Table 10.2. Characteristics of potential interventions to reduce transmission during Pandemic Alert Phases 5 and 6 and severe epidemics of seasonal influenza. (Reproduced with kind permission of the European Centre for Disease Prevention and Control (ECDC).)

Intervention	Quality of evidence[a]	Effectiveness (benefits)	Direct costs	Indirect costs and risks[b]	Acceptability	Practicalities and other issues
International travel (border closures, entry restrictions, travel advice)						
1. Travel advice	B	Minimal	Minimal	Massive	Good	International travel will probably decline massively anyway
2. Entry screening	B, Bm	Minimal	Moderate	Moderate	May be expected by resident population	Severe disruption at entry points. Many staff needed to screen travellers and implement follow-up action
3. Border closures or severe travel restrictions	B, Bm	Minimal unless almost complete	Massive	Massive	Variable, but may be expected by some in the resident populations	International travel will probably decline considerably anyway
Personal protective measures						
4. Regular hand washing	B	Probably reduces transmission	Minimal	Nil	Good, but compliance is unknown	Moderate[c], but requires targeted communication to maximize effectiveness
5. Good respiratory hygiene (use and disposal of tissues)	B	Unknown but presumed	Minimal	Minimal	Good, but compliance is unknown	Minimal, but requires targeted communication to maximize effectiveness
6. General mask wearing outside the home	C, Cm	Unknown	Massive	Minimal	Unknown, but little culture of mask wearing in many countries	Massive – difficulties of training, supply and types of masks, disposal and waste. May be perverse effects from misuse and re-use

A. Nicoll and H. Needham

7. Mask wearing in public settings (non-health)[d]	C	Unknown	Moderate	Minimal	Moderate – difficulties of training, defining high-risk situations, supply and types of mask
8. Mask wearing by people with respiratory infections	C	Unknown but presumed	Moderate	Minimal	Difficulties of defining those who should comply, and supply and types of mask. Also compliance for those with restricted breathing due to respiratory infection. May permit those ill and infectious to still circulate and infect others
9. Early self-isolation of ill people[e]	C	Unknown but presumed	Moderate	Moderate[f], will increase risk to carers and they will be off work	Need to train and equip home carers who will be at risk. Issue of compensation for lost wages and agreement of employers
10. Quarantine measures[g]	C	Unknown	Massive	Massive due to lost productivity	Very hard to make work equitably and issue of compensation for lost wages
Social distancing measures					
11. Internal travel restrictions	Cm, C	Minor delaying effect suggested	Moderate	Massive including social and economic disruption[h]	Key functions threatened. Issue of liability and legal basis[i]

continued

Table 10.2. Continued.

Intervention	Quality of evidence[a]	Effectiveness (benefits)	Direct costs	Indirect costs and risks[b]	Acceptability	Practicalities and other issues
12. Reactive school closures	Bm, C	May have greater effect than other social distancing	Moderate	Massive because of children needing to be cared for at home[j]	Unknown – does not happen often in most countries	Children out of school need to be kept away from other children (if not, epidemiological rationale is weakened). Issue of liability and legal basis[j,k]. Difficulties of timing, sustainability and re-opening
13. Proactive school closures	Bm, C	May have greater effect than other social distancing and be better than reactive	Moderate	As above[k]	As above	As above but even more difficulties of timing (may close too early), sustainability and re-opening[j,l]
14. Reactive workplace closures	Cm	Unknown[h]	Massive	Massive	Unknown, compensation issue crucial	Issue of liability, compensation and legal basis, also sustainability and re-opening. Not possible for key functions[l]
15. Home working and reducing meetings	Cm, C	Unknown	Moderate	Moderate	Likely to be acceptable	Less possible for key functions[m]
16. Cancelling public gatherings, international events, etc.	C	Unknown	Massive[h,i]	Massive[h,i]	Probably depends on compensation issue and if insurance applies[i]. May be expected by the public	Issue of liability and legal backing. Difficulty of definitions about what is a public gathering, international meeting and when to lift bans

Use of antivirals – early treatment

17. All those with symptoms	A (transmission and duration of illness only), Bm	Expected to be moderate but evidence on this limited[m]	Massive	Moderate	Expected by the public in most of the countries	Considerable logistical costs and difficulties in deciding who has influenza, delivering to all those who might benefit in a timely manner (under 24 or 48 h) and managing stocks equitably[n]
18. Health and social care and/or 'essential' workers	A	Minimal[o]	Moderate	Minimal	Considered part of staff protection and important for staff staying at work	Difficulties in defining who are health and social care workers or exposed key workers[o]

Use of antivirals – prophylaxis following a case

19. Family	B, Bm	Moderate	Massive	Moderate	Probably acceptable	Difficulties about case finding, defining families, speed of delivery, security and handling of stockpiles[o]
20. Family and other social contacts	B, Bm	Moderate	Massive+	Moderate	Unknown, but problem of people seemingly denied treatment	As above with problems of defining group boundaries
21. Family and geographical contacts	B, Bm	Moderate	Massive+	Moderate	Unknown, but problem of people seemingly denied treatment	As above with even more problems of defining group boundaries

continued

Table 10.2. Continued.

Intervention	Quality of evidence[a]	Effectiveness (benefits)	Direct costs	Indirect costs and risks[b]	Acceptability	Practicalities and other issues
Use of antivirals – continuous prophylaxis						
22. Health and social care and/or 'essential' workers	C	Moderate	Massive	Moderate	Unclear, health workers may not use them at all or not stay on them	Difficulties in defining who are health workers or essential workers. Issue of how long can keep offering antivirals
Vaccines – human–animal influenza vaccine ('pre-pandemic' vaccine)						
23. Whole population	B, Bm	Unclear, depends on cross-protection between vaccine subtype/strain and eventual wild-type pandemic virus[p]	Massive	Moderate[q]	Unknown[r,o]	Requires emphatic political support and much pre-planning. A phased approach may be needed
24. Health and social care workers and/or 'essential' workers	B, Bm	As above	Massive	As above	As above plus unclear that these groups will accept	As above. Difficulties in defining who are health/social care workers or essential workers
25. Children first	B, Bm	As above	Massive	As above	Especially unclear whether parents will accept, especially if disease is milder in children, benefit is for others and safety profile not well established[o]	As above. Needs pre-planning and parental support

Vaccines – specific pandemic vaccine

26. Pandemic-specific vaccines	B, Bm	Minimal in first wave	Massive and requires prior investment	Small	Probably highly acceptable°	Difficulty of deciding on initial priority groups

[a]Evidence of effectiveness: Grades A, B and C represent strongly, reasonably and poorly evidence-based recommendations, respectively. Grade A represents systematic reviews where there are diverse primary studies to draw from (not primarily modelling), well-designed epidemiological studies or especially experimental studies (randomized controlled trials). Grade B represents evidence based on well-designed epidemiological studies, substantial observational studies, experimental studies with five to 50 subjects or experimental studies with other limitations (like not having influenza as an endpoint). The code Bm indicates modelling work, with emphasis placed on studies that have available good-quality primary data. Hence quality can be both Bm and C. Grade C represents evidence based on case reports, small poorly controlled observational studies, poorly substantiated larger studies, application of knowledge of mode of transmission, infectiousness period, etc. Cm refers to modelling with few or poor-quality primary data.

[b]Sometimes called second-order and third-order effects, e.g. closing borders resulting in disruption of trade and movement of essential supplies and workers.

[c]Need to make frequent hand washing far more available and possible in daily settings, e.g. in public places, fast-food outlets, etc.

[d]People having face-to-face contact with many members of the public, in crowded travel settings.

[e]Usually at home of a person who is starting to feel unwell and feverish.

[f]Person requires care at home and they and their carers are lost from work.

[g]Isolation at home for some days of well people considered to have been exposed to infection.

[h]An advantage of this and some other interventions is that they will bring forward in a planned way what will probably happen anyway with time.

[i]Issue of who provides compensation if there is economic loss because of public (government) action.

[j]Child requires care at home and their carers are lost from work.

[k]Interventions targeted at children often assume they play an especially significant role in transmission, which may not be the case in every pandemic.

[l]There is a complex process of distinguishing what are and are not key functions, which is important but beyond the scope of this book.

[m]The evidence from trials is that with seasonal influenza early treatment reduces duration of illness and transmission. Estimates of the effect on hospitalization and mortality are observational, limited and far weaker.

[n]There is a series of major practical problems, e.g. deciding who has influenza, how to deliver the antivirals.

[o]There is a need to consider how early reports of plausible side-effects will be quickly and effectively investigated.

[p]Relies on assumptions about the strain type of the next pandemic. Benefit may be inferred from experimental serological responses, however, observational data and trials against the pandemic strain cannot be done before transmission starts and Phase 3. Trials may then be considered unethical.

[q]Financial risk that the next pandemic involves a different antigenic strain, i.e. a strain for which a vaccine has no cross-reactivity, and thus pre-pandemic vaccine is not effective.

[r]No country has offered population-wide vaccination with vaccine that may have low potential efficacy, hence major communication challenges.

that were applied or happened spontaneously in the three pandemics of the 20th century. These have revealed important and interesting observations. But these kinds of data can only generate hypotheses and suggestions; the evidence base is limited and primarily comprises anecdotal observations from the pandemics and seasonal outbreaks plus inferences from other scenarios and other respiratory infections, notably the outbreaks of severe acute respiratory syndrome (SARS) in 2003. There have been few field studies or trials of public health countermeasures during a pandemic, or even during seasonal epidemics, to evaluate their likely effectiveness and possible adverse secondary effects. Randomized control trials or randomized placebo-controlled trials (for pharmaceutical measures) might be desirable. However, many interventions simply cannot be trialled effectively because to do so would cause widespread disruption; and the conditions of a pandemic (novel virus and widespread population concern) cannot be adequately simulated in community trial settings. In the light of this, mathematical models have been used to project the possible impact of the interventions. Modelling is essential to investigate possible mechanisms and suggest what is more or less likely to happen (see Chapter 7).

Diversity in the characteristics and severity of pandemics

Pandemics are not standard (see Chapter 4). In particular they differ in:

- their severity – the impact on society including the proportion of infections that result in severe disease or death;
- the groups experiencing the most transmission and those most affected; and
- the influenza A subtype and phenotype, hence the likely effectiveness of pharmaceutical countermeasures.

These are crucial variables. The severity of a pandemic, whether it is mild, moderate or severe, will determine which public health measures can be justified. Measures like proactive closures of schools and cancellation of public events might be considered for a severe pandemic like that of 1918 but could be excessive for the milder pandemics of 1957, 1968 and 2009.

Similarly, if transmission is focused in one age band (as it was in 1957 in younger people) it may be worthwhile prioritizing measures that protect those age groups. However this would not have been so in 1968, when transmission was spread across all age groups. This emphasizes the need for early evaluation of the characteristics of pandemics, flexibility in the actions planned, national command and control structures that will allow rapid tailoring or even changing of strategies, and early evaluation of the effectiveness of specific measures where possible.

A further complication is that the characteristics of a pandemic will not be static. Pandemics change with time and as they spread, generally becoming less severe over time. This is because immunity develops in the population as the virus continues to evolve. Hence even if severity is found to be high in the early stages of a pandemic, it will be important to measure the epidemiological parameters at intervals, and in different settings, and to use this to assess which countermeasures could be usefully applied as the pandemic progresses.

A. Nicoll and H. Needham

Diversity within the pandemic

Influenza never affects all localities in the same way at the same time. This has been seen through the European Influenza Surveillance System (EISS) with seasonal influenza and will be equally true with a pandemic. Even if most places are eventually badly affected, this will not happen at the same time and this will have advantages and disadvantages. Given the patterns of spread seen with seasonal influenza in Europe (most commonly from west to east and south to north), it may be possible to give more warning to places in the north and east. Equally in countries with appropriate command and control structures it may be possible to move some healthcare resources (e.g. key staff, pharmaceuticals) around to relieve the most badly affected areas. However there are dangers and issues arising from the diversity of the pandemics (see next item). First, it will be a challenge for communicators to explain why certain measures are being enacted in one place but not another. Then with measures involving limited resources (antivirals, masks, etc.) care will be needed to ensure that supplies are not expended in the areas first affected leaving other populations with none when they are affected later.

The diversity of countries

It is self-evident that countries are highly diverse with varying population densities, social and legal frameworks both between and within countries. Hence a 'one size fits all' approach will not apply to some public health measures. Consider proactive early school closures – these may make particular sense in some dispersed rural areas and secondary schools where the schools are important foci for young people from scattered communities meeting together. However, they may make less sense and actually be counterproductive in dense urban areas where many parents may have to take time off work to care for children and where it will be difficult to stop children mixing anyway, out of school.

Isolated communities

Few places are sufficiently isolated that they will miss the pandemic. Although this was seen for a few places in the 1918 pandemic, the places that achieved this were exceptional and relatively self-sufficient. The world has become far more interconnected since the early 1900s and it is unlikely that more than a few per cent of citizens in Westernized countries live in communities that could self-isolate in this way.

Secondary effects

This concept, essentially looking at what are the costs, risks and consequences of applying the measures themselves, is crucial. The complexity underlying seemingly simple solutions to the pandemic threat such as 'close the borders' or 'close the schools' can be summarized in a famous saying attributed to the humorist H.L. Mencken: 'for every complex, difficult problem there is frequently a simple and attractive solution – that doesn't work'. Countermeasures, especially social distancing measures, almost certainly would have major unintended effects. Although they might reduce influenza transmission they might also be judged negative or unacceptable, certainly if it there has not been planning to overcome the secondary effects. For example, consider internal travel restrictions. These might slow or reduce transmission, but if it also means in highly interdependent societies that food or fuel supplies break down, they cannot be regarded a success. Equally, if schools are closed, it has to be determined who will look after the schoolchildren who are not at school. Will perhaps important staff (notably healthcare workers) be lost operationally because they have to take time off to look after their children? Public health countermeasures also have the potential to raise significant ethical issues relating to autonomy and curtailment of freedom. These are discussed in Chapter 12.

Timing of introduction and sustainability of countermeasures

It is a general principle with infectious diseases that early prevention is best. If countermeasures are to be applied, it is agreed that they generally need to be undertaken early in a pandemic if they are to be most effective. Overall, there is a suggestion from 1918 that public health measures instigated early tended to delay the peak in mortality by up to 2 weeks and reduce excess mortality. For example, it is suggested that proactive school closures (as the pandemic approaches) will be more effective in reducing transmission than reactive closures (waiting until cases occur in the school).

However, some of the measures will be difficult to sustain because of their secondary effects. If they are introduced too early the measures may break down as people grow frustrated with apparently pointless inhibitions to their daily lives and compliance wanes. Transmission then takes off again. There is historical evidence of this happening in the USA in the 1918 A/H1N1 pandemic, where a number of big cities attempted social distancing measures.

Focus Box 10.1. Some practicalities arising from school closures.

1. Educating, supervising and entertaining the children out of day care and school.
2. Negotiating leave (preferably paid) for parents/carers to enable them to be off work to care for children who are not sick.
3. Additional stress on those having to cover the work of those who are staying home with children.
4. Continuity of welfare and social programmes administered through schools.
5. The complexity of schools and school systems (public and private; state and religious based).
6. Defining the trigger points and timing for closure and re-opening of schools and geographic areas that would be involved given that a national system may not be desirable (see 'Diversity within the pandemic').
7. Defining practices for tertiary (university sector) education institutions with halls of residence, students whose homes are elsewhere in the country or even abroad and who may be 'trapped' at their college setting.
8. Communication with the staff, student body and families.
9. Meeting the needs of special groups, such as children with social disadvantages or learning/mental health difficulties.

A. Nicoll and H. Needham

Focus Box 10.2. **Modelling case study: travel restrictions.**

P.G. Grove, Senior Principal Analyst, Department of Health, Health Protection Analytical Team

When dealing with any pandemic, a natural response of an individual or community is to try to separate itself from the source of infection. Clearly, cutting a community off completely from the world would prevent infection reaching that community. However, in the modern world few countries are self-sufficient, particularly in terms of food, fuel and medical supplies. Only in a few special cases could a complete and indefinite 100% travel ban be put in place, and given this, would temporary or less complete restrictions help?

The limited usefulness of temporary restrictions of any kind is an immediate consequence of the epidemiological theory underlying any kind of model. As long as a large fraction of the community is susceptible, an epidemic will occur as soon as the first cases of the pandemic strain enter the country. The policy only makes sense if one can sustain the restrictions long enough for a pandemic-specific vaccine to become available in large quantities, i.e. for a period of at least 6 months after the beginning of the pandemic, but probably 1 year or more.

Could reducing the flow of people into a country or other community significantly delay arrival of the pandemic? Unfortunately, because influenza typically affects ten times as many people each 7–14 days, the reduction of initial cases entering the community by 90% would be expected to produce at best a 2-week delay in the epidemic in the community. Similarly a 99% reduction produces a 3- to 4-week delay, and 99.9% perhaps a couple of months.

These expectations have been confirmed by a number of explicit models of international travel[1], which also show more subtle effects. For example, with a cooperative policy where travel out of each community is reduced after the first few observed cases in that community, then the delay in the pandemic reaching other communities is twice that of similar universal entry restrictions imposed unilaterally by those communities.

The same argument backed up by explicit modelling also indicates that, given the period of approximately a day between infection and symptoms, neither exit or entry screening (for symptoms) is likely to be effective, producing only a few days' delay in the community's epidemic at most. The delay is even less if there is significant pre-symptomatic and asymptomatic transmission.

Similar arguments apply to travel within a larger community such as a country. Only very significant reductions (i.e. considerably more than half) in travel could be expected to make any significant difference to the spread of the national epidemic. Even then the effect would be to decouple the timing of 'local epidemics' in different parts of the country. Each local epidemic would put similar strain on the local health responders whether or not they were synchronized with other parts of the country.

In terms of the definitions of Chapter 7, travel restrictions are simply 'not robust over the range of uncertainty'.

[1]Cooper, B.S., Pitman, R.J., Edmunds, W.J. and Gay, N.J. (2006) Delaying the international spread of pandemic influenza. *PLoS Medicine* 3, 212.

Focus Box 10.3. Modelling case study: social distance measures and other non-pharmaceutical interventions.

P.G. Grove, Senior Principal Analyst, Department of Health, Health Protection Analytical Team

As stressed in Chapter 7, modelling is based on data. Its task is to make obvious that information which is not obvious in simply looking at the data used to construct the model. If there are no data, modelling can be of only limited value. Unfortunately, for many socially based interventions there are very little data and therefore little assistance available from modelling. A typical example is the value of the public use of face masks. There is currently no useful information on the effectiveness of face masks in reducing the transmission of influenza in the general community, and hence no data to put in a model. All that modelling can do here is say: 'we could buy N face masks which we have no information will save a single life, or we could use the same resources for an intervention which will avoid X deaths'.

Some information can be inferred on the possible effectiveness of social distance interventions by seeing if it is possible to model the epidemics in a number of American cities in the 1918 pandemic that adopted different social distance measures. Such an investigation was carried out by Bootsma and Ferguson[1]. They showed that it was indeed possible to fit models of interventions to the observed epidemic profiles for major cities. The most convincing evidence for the effectiveness of interventions was a second rise in the number of cases as interventions were relaxed. However, it is not clear if this provides useful information for policy formation. While a failure to explain the variation in terms of the interventions applied would be of interest, it is likely, given that we do not know how effective the interventions were, that some combination of assumptions about the interventions applied will in many cases be consistent with the observed data. The question is whether these assumptions are plausible. But this cannot easily be answered by fitting models to data.

The authors recommend caution in extrapolating from 1918 to the present day. Household sizes were much larger and many workers lived in large, crowded boarding houses within which transmission was probably intense. Far more people interacted with large extended families, children spent many fewer years in full-time education, and there were different travel patterns. Overall infectious disease mortality was much higher than it is today. Even taking the results at face value, the authors point out that to save substantial numbers of lives the measures need to be kept in place until there was enough vaccine to immunize the population. There would be huge social and economic consequences of imposing such measures for the many months that might be required for optimal effect.

The social measures that do have the most supporting information are school closures (at least for attending pupils). Even here the effectiveness of closing schools depends critically on how children are assumed to mix with other children and adults. A wide range of impacts has been claimed in the literature. The UK government's Scientific Pandemic Influenza Advisory Group (SPI)[2] considers the most credible results come from studies based on school holidays in the UK and France[3].

continued

A. Nicoll and H. Needham

Focus Box 10.3. Continued.

These indicate that school closures are most effective at reducing illness in school-children. The total effect on the number of clinical cases in the entire population is little more than one-tenth (in the range of 10–20%) although the reduction in peak incidence could be higher, up to 50%. Although of limited value themselves, school closures are a very effective adjunct to a household prophylactic approach using antiviral drugs (see Chapter 8). It is important to take into account when estimating the effect of school closures the fact that children may not stay at home if schools are closed and this would reduce the effectiveness of the policy.

Closing schools in countries like the UK has the potential to create large amounts of absenteeism from work, as working parents would have to stay at home to look after their children. The UK SPI estimates that such absenteeism could be as high as 17–20% of the workforce, similar to that expected directly from illness at the peak of the epidemic.

[1]Bootsma, M.C. and Ferguson, N.M. (2007) The effect of public health measures on the 1918 influenza pandemic in US cities. *Proceedings of the National Academy of Sciences USA* 104, 7588–7593.
[2]UK Scientific Pandemic Influenza Committee (SPI) *Subgroup on Modelling (2008) Modelling Summary*. http://www.advisorybodies.doh.gov.uk/spi/minutes/spi-m-modellingsummary.pdf (accessed May 2009).
[3]Cauchemez, S., Valleron, A.J., Boëlle, P.Y., Flahault, A. and Ferguson, N.M. (2008) Estimating the impact of school closure on influenza transmission from sentinel data. *Nature* 452, 750–755.

Dealing with the first outbreaks

A difficult issue is what to do when the first outbreak occurs in a country during WHO Pandemic Alert Phase 5 or 6. In some simulation exercises, a number of authorities have tried to contain the first outbreaks using conventional measures (such as contact tracing) and distributing large amounts of antivirals to ring-fence the outbreaks by treating patients and prophylaxing their contacts. The scenarios have always been that the measures seem to have delayed spread a little, but have failed to contain the infection. In addition, resources have been expended and public health staff exhausted before the pandemic has really started. There are also difficulties in explaining to professionals and the public any antiviral policy switch from treatment and prophylaxis (in the early stages) to treatment only (as the pandemic takes hold).

Complete protection or mitigation?

Many of the measures in this chapter are not expected or even intended to give complete protection. They will mitigate or reduce the risk, but not eliminate it; they are a public health approach to reduce the overall impact on the population. This is especially important with the measures that have significant secondary effects, where complete implementation may be unacceptable. That is why some governments would intend to apply not one but a number of measures. However, given the nature of infection and pandemics there are some measures where only almost complete implementation would be effective, notably those intended to totally block entry of the virus into a population (e.g. border closures). In these cases the intervention may have greater negative consequences than the disease itself.

Layered containment measures – 'defence in depth'

Current thinking is that the impact of any single public health measure will be limited because they are hard to enact and do not work perfectly, indeed some may fail entirely. By applying a number of countermeasures simultaneously there will be a cumulative effect on transmission. Some have argued that given the relatively low infectivity of influenza it may be possible to prevent transmission chains building up or to interrupt transmission, however, that assumes a cumulative effect of the measures, which is currently a theoretical concept. There is some encouragement for this view from the experience when SARS cases were occurring in Hong Kong in 2003. Multiple measures were enacted by the authorities (including closing schools, forbidding public events) or just happened because they made sense to the citizens (such as staying home and wearing masks when people went out). This is not thought to be what ultimately controlled SARS, but there was a coincidental significant impact on influenza incidence as reflected in laboratory reports. However, there are also important considerations of cumulative costs and secondary effects with multiple measures, i.e. not only the benefits will increase, but so also will the adverse effects.

The necessity of intersectoral planning and preparation

Intersectoral planning and preparation is crucial for many of the public health measures. If regular hand washing is important, there need to be facilities in schools and public places to enable this. If it is thought that masks will be needed for some workers, these will need to be ordered by employers. Actions involving schools will need preparation not just by educational authorities, private and public schools, but also other sectors, industry and civil society. If parents have to seek other care for their children, they cannot be in groups or the purpose of the closures will be undermined. If they have to take time off work is it agreed that they will be paid?

Legal issues and liability

Enacting some of the public health measures require legal powers and obviously this has to be planned for. There is also the complex area of who is liable for any financial loss that can be said to be due to the measures versus the pandemic. This is genuinely difficult. For example, if it is thought that an international or national meeting should be cancelled, should this be a decision by the authorities who may then be financially liable or is it better to wait until it is clear that many people are cancelling in which case the organizers will have to cancel themselves? These considerations can prevent early action even when it is desirable.

A. Nicoll and H. Needham

General versus selective measures

General measures (such as everyone wearing masks, everyone taking antivirals) have simplicity and equity. However, they may not make sense to people who perceive obvious variation in risk and therefore are less acceptable than selective measures for those at higher risk (e.g. people exposed to the general public wearing masks). Selective measures allow more possibilities for ensuring quality in the application of the measure and can allow more efficient use of supplies. However the recurrent issues with selective measures are boundaries and policing, deciding who should practise measures and who should not, and preventing people feeling left out of benefiting from measures or getting anxious or annoyed that some people seem to be breaking the rules.

Early recognition and diagnosis

A number of the measures (e.g. early use of antivirals) will require early recognition and diagnosis of influenza as infectivity is considered greatest within a day after onset of symptoms, and children and people with disabilities will need special consideration. It must be appreciated that this will not be by laboratory test. There will not be the time, laboratories will be too busy and the point-of-use (bed-side) tests may not work with the new pandemic strain of virus. Hence much of the diagnosis will be presumptive by signs and symptoms alone.

Communications

The importance of this for the public health measures cannot be over-emphasized. All the measures require close cooperation by the public, professionals and decision makers. Communication materials explaining them will need to be prepared ahead of time, pre-tested and probably re-written. Equally there will need to be surge capacity in communication specialists for the pandemic as there is for other key staff (Chapter 13).

Special groups – special considerations

There will be a number of groups who will find it especially difficult to comply with measures, such as the elderly (especially those living alone), children, homeless people or those living in poverty or institutions, people travelling but 'caught' in another country, people with physical or learning difficulties, and those with special communication needs (e.g. hearing difficulties, visually impaired, not speaking the national languages). In some cases numbers will be substantial and planning will need to take this into account.

Protective sequestration – children and adolescents

It was suggested by some authorities that early in a pandemic children and adolescents should be prevented from congregating in groups by closing childcare facilities and schools and requiring them to stay at home for the local duration of a pandemic (3–4 months). This might be possible in some settings but not in most and, after some thought, no country has considered this as a serious option for a mass intervention.

Work quarantine

This is where quarantine is observed or special measures are taken by health or social care workers who have been exposed *and* who work in settings where influenza is especially liable to transmit (or where there are people at higher risk from infection). Examples would be people working in old people's homes and nurses in high-risk settings (such as neonatal care nurseries or intensive care units). This practice was quite common during the SARS crisis but has far less relevance during a pandemic, where, paradoxically, the threat of infection will be prevalent throughout society and not just in the healthcare environment.

Interoperability

This multifaceted term has a number of meanings – both positive and negative (Table 10.3). For example, neighbouring states or regions need to consider the impact of enacting public health measures on their neighbours, such as closing borders if that stops movement of essential workers. Because of modern communications there can also be indirect effects through the media if one state is seen enacting measures such as screening entrants or mask wearing.

There are also positive aspects of interoperability, for example, if a few countries work for the benefit of all. There is a strong tradition of this in the influenza field,

Table 10.3. National and international interoperability and pandemic planning.

Negative	Positive
A country does something that impacts negatively direct on your state, e.g. closing borders if that stops daily commuting for work	Some countries perform work from which all (or neighbours) benefit. Actions that can be undertaken most efficiently in a few MS rather than all MS but of benefit to all, e.g. monitoring for the development of antiviral resistance
A country does something that causes questions in another state – especially if it is done without warning, e.g. starting publicly screening people coming off flights	A group of countries share thinking and analyses on particular policy areas so that conclusions emerge from a common understanding of what is known and not known, e.g. whether and when to close schools proactively
	Countries share experience and development while recognizing their differences (one size will not fit all)
	A country talks specifically with its immediate neighbours in relation to all the above
	A country warns all others as to what it plans to do in a pandemic
	International bodies like ECDC and WHO develop common mechanisms and tools for preparing and dealing with pandemics, e.g. the ECDC Pandemic Preparedness Assessment Tool

MS, member state; ECDC, European Centre for Disease Prevention and Control; WHO, World Health Organization.

A. Nicoll and H. Needham

with a limited number of WHO Collaborating Centres serving to do specialist virology for the world. Work such as measuring the likely antiviral resistance, determining case fatality rates and the effectiveness of antivirals could, for example, be efficiently spread around Europe rather than duplicated in all 27 EU Member States. There has also been careful thinking about the public health measures themselves in a number of States. If more of this is done collectively on particular policy areas, then knowledge and work can be shared and conclusions emerge from a common understanding of what is known and not known. Even if states eventually come to different decisions (e.g. on whether to purchase human A/H5N1 vaccines and whether and when to close schools proactively) at least it will be done on a common basis.

10.6 Summary Points

- Countermeasures can be defined as group actions taken that are intended to reduce human-to-human transmission of influenza and by that way mitigate the adverse effects of a pandemic. Some actions are really individual actions designed to give personal protection (e.g. hand washing, mask wearing) or even treatment (e.g. taking of antiviral drugs and use of vaccines) but when taken en masse can result in overall reductions in transmission and so have a public health benefit.

- Many of the measures would have some impact in terms of reducing transmission although they are less than might at first be imagined, because even if influenza is stopped by one route or in one setting it will come though another. The greatest impact may therefore be through using multiple measures. Then the effects may be additive, but so will be the costs.

- The potential costs, secondary effects, risks and practical experience of the suggested countermeasures vary. Some are minor (routine hand washing), others are massive (school closures); none is trivial. In some cases the negative effects will greatly outweigh the gains.

- The same countermeasures cannot necessarily be applied in all circumstances. Each pandemic studied so far has had some distinct features. Nevertheless, there will need to be default sets of recommended public health measures. Also, because of different circumstances in different countries, the measures will not be the same in every country.

- It is difficult to determine which of the suggested measures is likely to be most helpful and which the least, as this depends on the circumstances and the pandemic. Also there are many measures where we are simply not sure of their effectiveness. However, there are some that we know will not be effective in a pandemic or they are simply impractical – such as measures at borders like trying to screen people (does not work) or sealing borders (usually impractical).

Acknowledgements

The chapter authors and book editors wish to acknowledge that this chapter has been written with the full support of the European Centre for Disease Prevention and Control (ECDC). The chapter draws upon the paper *ECDC Background Advice on Public Health Measures that may be Deployed in the Event of an Influenza Pandemic or Severe Epidemics of Seasonal Influenza – version October 2007* available at http://ecdc.europa.eu/en/Health_Topics/Pages/Pandemic_Influenza_Public_Health_ Measures.aspx (accessed June 2009).

Further Reading

Cooper, B.S., Pitman, R.J., Edmunds, W.J. and Gay, N.J. (2006) Delaying the international spread of pandemic influenza. *PLoS Medicine* 3, 212.

Cauchemez, S., Valleron, A.J., Boëlle, P.Y., Flahault, A. and Ferguson, N.M. (2008) Estimating the impact of school closure on influenza transmission from sentinel data. *Nature* 452, 750–755.

Cauchemez, S., Ferguson, N.M., Watchtel, C., Tegnell, A., Saour, G., Duncan, B. and Nicoll, A. (2009) Closure of schools during an influenza pandemic. *Lancet Infectious Diseases* 9, 473–481.

European Centre for Disease Prevention and Control (2009) *Guide to public health measures to reduce the impact of influenza pandemics in Europe – The ECDC Menu.* http://ecdc. europa.eu/en/publications/Publications/0906_TER_Public_Health_Measures_for_ influenza_pandemics.pdf (accessed May 2009).

Ferguson, N.M., Cummings, D.A., Fraser, C., Cajka, J.C., Cooley, P.C. and Burke, D.S. (2006) Strategies for mitigating an influenza pandemic. *Nature* 442, 448–452.

Inglesby, T.V., Nuzzo, J.B., O'Toole, T. and Henderson, D.A. (2006) Disease mitigation measures in the control of pandemic influenza. *Biosecurity and Bioterrorism: Biodefense Strategy, Practice and Science* 4(4), 1–10.

Markel, H., Lipman, H.B., Navarro, J.A., Sloan, A., Michalsen, J.R., Stern, A.M. and Cetron, M.S. (2007) Non-pharmaceutical interventions implemented by US cities during the 1918–1919 influenza pandemic. *Journal of the American Medical Association* 298, 644–654. Erratum in *Journal of the American Medical Association* 2007, 298, 2264.

World Health Organization (2006) *WHO pandemic influenza draft protocol for rapid response and containment*, Updated draft 30 May 2006. http://www.who.int/csr/disease/avian_ influenza/guidelines/protocolfinal30_05_06a.pdf (accessed May 2009).

World Health Organization (2007) Epidemic and Pandemic Alert and Response (EPR). *WHO Interim Protocol: Rapid operations to contain the initial emergence of pandemic influenza.* Updated October 2007. http://www.who.int/csr/disease/avian_influenza/guidelines/ draftprotocol/en/index.html (accessed May 2009).

World Health Organization (2009) *Epidemic and Pandemic Alert and Response (EPR). Pandemic influenza prevention and mitigation in low resource communities.* 2 May 2009. http://www.who.int/csr/resources/publications/swineflu/low_resource_measures/en/ index.html (accessed June 2009).

A. Nicoll and H. Needham

11 Societal and Economic Impacts of an Influenza Pandemic

R. PULESTON

- Should pandemic planning focus on healthcare provision alone?
- How might non-health businesses be affected by the pandemic?
- Can we learn from other events?
- What is the potential financial impact of a pandemic?
- In the next pandemic what will be the causes of workplace absenteeism?

11.1 Introduction

Influenza pandemics have occurred throughout history. The scientific community has commented that it is only a matter of time before another is experienced. What will be the impact of such an event on the societal and economic fabric of the global society? This chapter explores some of the possible effects of a future pandemic on societal functioning.

Much will depend on the virulence and rapidity of spread of the emergent virus and the response taken by governments and the public. Previous pandemics have been very variable in impact. Unfortunately, only limited data are available on which to form predictions because pandemics are relatively infrequent events. The best data emanate from the three pandemics that occurred in the 20th century (1918, 1957 and 1968). The two latter events had a (numerically) relatively small impact on mortality although they did cause considerable increases in demand for healthcare services. The 1918 outbreak was at the other end of the spectrum with widespread disruption and substantial global mortality. What will be the impact of the next pandemic? It is impossible to say with any certainty, however, there are key changes to global society that will shape the event. These will be explored in this chapter.

The uncertainties around the possible impact of future influenza pandemics make planning and preparedness very difficult. While on one hand there is the potential to be accused of scaremongering, on the other if a serious outbreak does occur, questions will inevitably be asked as to why more action was not taken before the event. To quote the former US Health and Human Services Secretary, Michael O. Leavitt: 'Everything you say in advance of a pandemic is alarmist; anything you do after it starts is inadequate'.

11.2   Human Health Impacts

Mortality

Seasonal influenza exacts a toll every year, mainly on the old and infirm. Those with underlying conditions such as respiratory problems or reduced immune systems are more likely to succumb to the disease. For example, in the USA, some 36,000 die annually during the season as a result of the infection, while in the UK there is an average of 12,000 excess deaths annually attributed to seasonal influenza.

However, while it is anticipated that the mortality experienced during a pandemic could be orders of magnitude greater, history is not very consistent on this. The 1918 pandemic produced a high mortality globally, 20–40 million people worldwide are thought to have died with some estimates placing this figure nearer 100 million. The events later in the century had a much smaller mortality impact, thought to be in the region of one million excess deaths, not vastly different from the annual global death toll attributed to seasonal influenza.

The variability of mortality makes it very difficult to predict with any precision what will be experienced in a future pandemic. Nevertheless, governments around the world have planned for a pandemic that could realize deaths in the upper range of that previously experienced in 1918. For example, the UK government has planned for a reasonable worst case scenario of 50% clinical attack rate and a case fatality rate of up to 2.5%. The World Health Organization (WHO) predicted a global mortality from the next pandemic of about 7.4 million, while World Bank estimates in 2006 placed the expected mortality at up to 1.08% of the global population or approximately 72 million people. Some researchers have suggested that the figures may be substantially higher at 250 million deaths.

What is known from the last century is that the spike in deaths caused major problems with dealing with the dead, particularly so in 1918. Undertakers and burial authorities were overwhelmed by the numbers of deceased. As a consequence, planners are considering how they might respond should similar circumstances occur again, spanning from streamlining death certification processes to managing the high demand for funeral services.

Conventional seasonal influenza tends to afflict the very young, the elderly and those with weak immune systems or certain chronic diseases. This was also experienced with the two milder pandemics of 1957 and 1968. However, the 1918 pandemic behaved differently. While the first wave conformed to this usual pattern, the second saw large numbers of working-age adults (aged 20–45 years) killed with relative sparing of the very young and old. The reasons for this are not fully understood.

Morbidity

With up to 50% of the population being affected by symptomatic influenza over the course of an influenza pandemic, it is clear that the potential for disruption due to the ill health that ensues will be substantial. While it is expected that most illness will

R. Puleston

be self-limiting and relatively minor, there will be a minority who become more severely ill. The less badly affected are nevertheless predicted to be absent from work for approximately 5–10 days due to the illness itself.

US estimates have indicated that approximately one-sixth of the population (17%) will seek 'outpatient' care and about 0.7%–3% will require hospital care, with up to 0.5% needing intensive-level care. Other estimates suggest that of those who become infected with symptoms, up to 25% will need medical help, with between 0.55% and 4% needing hospital treatment and up to 1% warranting intensive care.

Typically influenza causes respiratory symptoms (cough) and fever. However, it can cause a range of other symptoms – including neurological (encephalopathy), muscular (myositis) and abdominal (diarrhoea) effects (Chapter 1). Viral pneumonia has a high mortality and can be additionally complicated by secondary bacterial infection. Until the epidemiological characteristics of the emergent virus are clear, it will remain uncertain what symptoms will be predominant. Additionally, individuals with existing co-morbidities (e.g. asthma, heart disease and chronic obstructive pulmonary disease) are more likely to be adversely affected.

Psychiatric morbidity

Mass casualty/fatality events are known to produce significant psychiatric morbidity for the surviving victims, relatives and friends, and rescuing staff. Perhaps less clear in contemporary times are the effects of an event of much larger magnitude, including an influenza pandemic. The 9/11 terrorist attacks in New York in 2001, the Indian Ocean tsunami of December 2004 and the effect of Hurricane Katrina on New Orleans, USA in 2005 can give some pointers.

These events have and will continue to have profound effects on the survivors (direct and indirect) and their mental health, but will most likely be dwarfed by a future pandemic. Risk factors for an adverse mental health outcome include multiple intense stressors, bereavement, threat to life, financial loss and displacement. Additionally, there is some evidence that victims in developing countries possibly fare less well than those in developed nations.

Health systems will need to be prepared to respond to the psychological needs of survivors, but this will have to be carefully managed to ensure effective support, otherwise further harm may ensue.

11.3 Financial Costs

The financial costs of an influenza pandemic could be enormous – modelling has suggested that they could be in the region of several trillions of US dollars. The costs will be felt across society, from increased healthcare provision requirements, through lost productivity of industry, to early deaths and short- and long-term disability of victims of the outbreak. However, it is not only these expenditures immediately associated with a pandemic that should be borne in mind. The financial outlay made in preparation for a pandemic is ongoing and substantial. This poses significant dilemmas for planners in terms of the opportunity costs of making these investments. Post-pandemic recovery costs will also be considerable.

It is probable that emerging economies will be more adversely affected financially. In emergency situations, investors tend to switch to safe havens and thus a flight of capital to lower-risk assets is possible.

The pandemics of the 20th century can be broadly categorized into severe, moderate and mild in terms of their overall impact. A recent report by Lloyds of London Insurance assessed the possible impact on the international economy as ranging from a 1% to a 10% reduction in gross domestic product (GDP). It goes on to suggest that although a pandemic of 1918 levels is looked upon as the 'worst case scenario', this should not be assumed to be the worst possible level of impact.

The financial consequences of an influenza pandemic are expected to vary by country, region and industry type. Those more dependent on tourism, travel and entertainment are likely to be hit hardest with GDP reductions of up to 8%, whereas those with more diverse economies will probably fare better with GDP decreases of up to approximately 5%.

In 2006 the World Bank estimated that the cost of an influenza pandemic could be as much as US$2 trillion or 3.2% GDP reduction. News reports indicate that it has since revised the figure to US$3 trillion (the world economy therefore being worth approximately US$60 trillion annually) or a 4.8% GDP decline, with lower levels estimated for less severe attacks of between 0.7% and 2% of GDP (US$400 billion to US$1.2 trillion).

The direct costs of a pandemic are only a small proportion of the economic impact. It is expected that by trying to avoid infection, the resultant behaviour changes will cause 60% of the predicted economic losses. The experience with severe acute respiratory syndrome (SARS) provides some useful parallels here. The number of deaths was relatively small and yet the losses due to people trying to avoid infection were substantial. The World Bank estimates that the financial losses that will occur due to deaths and infection are, respectively, only 20% and 40% of the cost of anticipated behavioural changes.

Estimating the potential impact a pandemic might have on the economy of a country is fraught with the same problems that all aspects of pandemic planning face – the large number of unknowns. The UK government has calculated that the potential financial impact to that country due to illness-related absence from work could reduce the year's GDP by between £3 and £7 billion. The excess deaths caused by the pandemic could result in a further reduction of between £1 and £7 billion in the pandemic year. The variance comes from the uncertainty around the case fatality rate and whether earnings or gross output are calculated. In the longer term, further calculations can be made around the financial impact of the premature deaths due to a pandemic, taking into account assumptions about the age ranges of those affected by the pandemic and future economic trends. The potential reduction in future lifetime earnings could range from £21 to £26 billion at a low case fatality rate and from £145 to £172 billion at a high case fatality rate.

R. Puleston

Post-event litigation and enquiries

Lloyds of London has commented that organizations that effectively plan and test their arrangements for an influenza pandemic are less likely to be involved in litigation after the event. Despite this, it appears that only a small proportion of companies (mainly large ones) have made preparations or contingency arrangements to deal with the threat (Chapter 6).

Professionals are rightly concerned that, despite acting in good faith before and during a pandemic, they may be taken to task afterwards for their actions. Regulators, professional bodies, legal authorities and governments need to include and act on these concerns in their preparations.

Actions by individuals, organizations or companies may come under scrutiny once the pandemic is over. Insurance claims are likely to climb after a pandemic, for example from cancelled travel or events and insured business losses. Organizations can mitigate some of these possibilities by carefully assessing the risks they face and planning appropriately for them.

11.4 Industrial Impacts

Modelling has suggested that an influenza pandemic will cause industrial output to decline to a level consistent with the recessions that have occurred since the end of World War II. Some sectors of the economy are likely to face bigger declines than others. In particular, mass transport, restaurants, large entertainment gatherings and hotels will probably be affected most. The World Bank estimates that the SARS outbreak led to an overall decline of 0.5% in the GDP of the East Asian economy, with a steeper decline of 2% in the second quarter of 2003 when publicity about the disease was at its peak. This provides some indication of what may happen during an influenza pandemic, however, it is important to bear in mind that the SARS outbreak was of much smaller scale than an influenza pandemic will be.

Governments around the world are working on the presumption of maintaining business and services towards as normal a state of affairs as possible because to advise otherwise would risk causing even greater harm. The virulence of the outbreak will determine whether this is achievable. If mild it may not be difficult to persuade people to continue to work, but if severe many may consider the risks as too great for them. Management of the perceived risks will be important as people are not always good at determining the degree of threat they face, which can lead to inappropriate responses. Businesses should make preparations for an influenza pandemic to enable them to maintain their services and protect their staff during the crisis. Many large, international businesses will have done this, especially financial institutions, but this work needs to be undertaken by small and medium-sized companies too in all business sectors (Chapter 6).

An examination of some of the press reports from the time of the 1918 outbreak reveals that some businesses were affected quite badly through absenteeism. For example, the output of some mining companies reduced and was attributed to widespread illness in the workers. The City of London Stock Exchange was reported at the time to have been disrupted by traders being unable to attend for business, such that the effect on financial liquidity required intervention by the Bank of England.

While many businesses will be negatively impacted during a pandemic, others may see a surge in demand. As people choose to stay away from crowded areas, there may be an increase in online shopping for groceries – will companies have sufficient transport to deliver food to their customers? There will inevitably be a demand for over-the-counter healthcare products and cleaning products among the general public, and companies will need to ensure they can manufacture and supply enough to meet demand.

Absenteeism

Work absence during an influenza pandemic is likely to be determined by the severity of the outbreak, the degree of concern generated and the subsequent public response. It will be affected to varying degrees throughout the pandemic.

By definition, if the attack rate is either 25 or 50%, then over the course of the pandemic it is likely that 25–50% of staff will not attend work for a period of time. More problematic to predict are the possible levels of absence at the peak of the pandemic wave. Estimates vary from 10 to 30% of the working population or between a doubling and a two-thirds increase in absence levels in the private and public sector, respectively. This will vary by industry type, with health and social care likely to have a greater problem than for example goods distribution because of the larger potential for exposure to the infection. Some of the non-attendance will be due to caring responsibilities (either through sickness or school closure), transport disruptions and also possible work avoidance due to fear of catching the virus either at work or on the way to work.

Employers may already be developing staffing contingency plans for an influenza pandemic. Some businesses/organizations may still have to make such arrangements. This is more likely to be the case in smaller establishments, but as they can make up a large part of the economy, it is particularly important that they too consider how they would continue to staff their business during an influenza pandemic.

Enabling staff to work at home, away from their normal office, is a sensible measure to take; however, as the number of people working remotely rises, an increasing demand will be made on telecommunications networks – both telephone and Internet.

Resources

Much of the industrialized world has, for sound commercial reasons, moved towards lean business methods where costs are restrained by reducing stock levels to the minimum possible and instead receiving replenishment on a 'just in time' basis. While this makes sense during normal operating conditions, it unfortunately increases vulnerability to supply chain interruptions. The implications of this are that when a disruptive event occurs, supplies may become vulnerable, due to either rapid increases

R. Puleston

in demand for particular goods that cannot be easily met owing to insufficient capacity to scale up rapidly or the logistic network itself breaking down and becoming unable to maintain normal deliveries. These are both possible during an influenza pandemic of sufficient magnitude.

Consumables

As the pandemic threat starts to increase, there is likely to be a sudden surge in demand for certain types of supply, in particular personal protective equipment, healthcare equipment and some pharmaceuticals. Most countries import at least some of these items and therefore have little direct control over the maintenance of supply. Prices are likely to rise under these circumstances. Those countries with the deepest pockets will be best able to access these scarce resources, leaving poorer areas more vulnerable to being unable to fulfil their needs.

Once the pandemic gets underway for real, the subsequent effects on supply chains will depend on how severe it is. If, after the initial rush for stocking essential supplies, the emerging epidemiology indicates a probable mild attack, then demand may decline again. If, however, it is severe, requirements will continue to rise through the wave and it is possible as a result that some countries may adopt a protectionist stance to preserve stocks for domestic consumption. Some regions will experience the onset of the pandemic earlier than others and therefore may be better placed to get in supplies early, while those affected later may have more difficulties.

Pharmaceuticals

Several specific examples of where supplies may come under particular pressure are influenza vaccines, antiviral drugs and antibiotics. Routine seasonal influenza vaccine manufacturing facilities will have to be diverted to the production of pandemic-specific vaccines. Seasonal vaccine manufacturing has little in the way of spare capacity after meeting the annual demand for seasonal vaccine. Only a proportion of the countries around the world have annual influenza vaccination programmes. While the existing manufacturers can switch their facilities to produce a pandemic-specific vaccine, the capacity would not be sufficient to meet the needs of the entire global population by some considerable degree. Therefore there will be delays and shortages in the supply of the vaccine (Chapter 9).

Likewise, antiviral drugs specific to treating influenza and antibiotics to treat secondary bacterial respiratory infections will be in high demand. The antiviral drugs specific to treating influenza do not have much routine demand out of the seasonal influenza season and therefore manufacturing capacity would otherwise under normal commercial rules be restricted. However, some countries have made efforts to stockpile antiviral drugs in preparation for a pandemic occurring, so availability is better than it otherwise might have been. While in normal times antibiotics are in fairly constant demand (some seasonal winter increase) and manufacturing capacity covers that 'steady state' requirement, this is not likely to be the case during a pandemic. Some countries are now starting to consider antibiotic stockpiling as the capacity to respond to an increase in requirements will be difficult to meet without prior planning (Chapter 8).

Fuel and food

Somewhat paradoxically, a severe pandemic would in some respects be more challenging for highly industrialized countries than those countries still developing because the 'life support systems' of the former are highly integrated and interdependent. Food, utilities and other essential supplies are all vital to maintain the population. Any significant disruption to such systems would be rapidly felt. Contrast this with more rural, self-sustaining communities already used to having to fend for themselves, who will perhaps be in a better position to cope. Authorities in the former therefore need to emphasize the maintenance of 'business as much as usual' as is possible during the pandemic.

Travel

During the SARS outbreak of 2003, international travel to the affected areas declined markedly. The WHO advised against non-essential travel to those areas and people also voluntarily reduced their flying. A similar pattern would probably be seen during an influenza pandemic and it is likely that people will be advised against non-essential travel. However, modelling has suggested that restricting travel compulsorily would not significantly delay the spread of the disease internationally. Some countries may nevertheless close their borders. Border screening was not found to have been helpful during the SARS outbreak and is therefore unlikely to be recommended. Domestic travel restrictions for similar reasons would probably not be helpful. However, people using public transport will probably be advised to stagger their journeys.

11.5 Societal Maintenance and Breakdown

What will be the impact of an influenza pandemic on normal social functioning? The experience of previous disasters can give an indication. The pandemic of 1918 did see considerable difficulties, but press reports at the time indicate that in the large part people continued about their normal daily lives as best they could. The population as a whole continued to go to work/school, banks and businesses continued to open. In short, there was no meltdown of society.

Contrast that with the aftermath of Hurricane Katrina in 2005, where New Orleans very rapidly collapsed into a reported state of semi-anarchy. Food, water, utilities and other essential supplies became scarce or unavailable. Law and order broke down in some parts of the city. There were also reports of some essential service workers abandoning their responsibilities.

R. Puleston

Probably the essential difference between the two examples above was the speed with which the disaster struck. The former developed slowly and presumably allowed time for the public to adapt. It was also at a time of difficult circumstances for many, coming at the end of World War I and in a different era, which may have modified expectations, attitudes and behaviours. In contrast, Hurricane Katrina hit with relatively little notice and caused a rapid disintegration of the infrastructure of the city to which the residents had little time to adjust and prepare for. Changes in societal cohesiveness may have also had effects on the population's reaction. Cultural differences may also be of relevance in between-country responses. A new influenza pandemic is therefore likely to have different social manifestations across the globe.

Legal issues, civil unrest and illegal activity

There are numerous legal issues to be considered in planning for a possible influenza pandemic. These will vary from country to country dependent on their legal systems. However, in broad terms some of the questions to potentially consider include emergency powers, certification of death, rationing of scarce resources including healthcare, prescribing and public health control measures. Each country will need to review its own legislation to assess if changes are required to meet the demands of an influenza pandemic.

Healthcare staff may have concerns over their legal and regulatory protection during a pandemic. For example, there may be worries that in the course of making difficult decisions during the outbreak, they may be criticized or face legal action after the event. In order to retain staff confidence, it is important they feel reassured that provided they act in good faith and to professional standards appropriate to the situation, they will not get into difficulties subsequently. Governments and regulatory authorities are working on this is some countries, but others may still need to do so. This may include ensuring that indemnity insurance arrangements and regulatory approval arrangements are adequate and in place for existing staff, displaced staff, volunteers and voluntary agencies/charities.

One of the consequences of crises is the potential for civil unrest and illegal activity, which was seen particularly in the wake of Hurricane Katrina and the tsunami in 2004. Looting and other criminality were widely reported in the aftermath of the disaster in New Orleans. There were fewer reports of problems of this nature after the tsunami, although perhaps the huge mortality and massive disruption focused attention elsewhere. A concern of planners in the context of influenza preparations is that if there are large numbers of ill people trying to access healthcare facilities, there could be the potential for control to break down. Where countries have stockpiled resources, such as antiviral medications, security will be an issue. Preparations therefore need to include how staff, facilities and resources can be protected under these sorts of circumstances. In emergency situations, the humanitarian response of volunteering to help may come to the fore. Unfortunately, some unscrupulous individuals may use the opportunity to exploit the vulnerable. This possibility needs to be guarded against.

Prisons and other closed institutions

The management of cases occurring in prisons and other closed institutions such as barracks, secure mental health units and boarding schools presents particular problems during major infectious disease outbreaks. The confined nature of these premises can facilitate efficient spread of infection, leading to potentially large numbers of people becoming ill in a short space of time. Where reasonable worst case scenario planning may put the general community infection rate at 50% of the population, in a closed community such as a prison this could rise to 90% of individuals. Providing healthcare under these circumstances may be challenging. Where security is also an issue, especially for prisons and secure mental health units and where the population cannot be dispersed for safety reasons, management of pandemic influenza will be even more challenging.

During an influenza pandemic, estimates indicate that approximately 4% of those afflicted may need hospital-level treatment, of which a quarter may need intensive-level care. In a closed institution it is likely that the numbers will be higher. Providing hospital-level care to those who need it under these circumstances will be very difficult. For secure units, transfers to acute hospitals may be complicated or impossible if security cannot be provided (due to the numbers involved or loss of staff) and yet the facilities and available staff may not be equipped or skilled to deal with patients who are severely ill on site.

Solutions are not easy, but must be planned and exercised in advance. Quarantining prisons, barracks or mental health units to prevent influenza entering the facility may be an option, but would have severe knock-on consequences for the normal functioning of the services that rely on these institutions. Shifting healthcare resources including staff and equipment into a prison, for example, may be required. Alternatively (and this may difficult for the wider public to accept), the occupants of these institutions may have to be prioritized for treatment and/or prophylaxis with antiviral drugs and immunization against influenza with a pandemic-specific vaccine.

Schools and education

Children are efficient spreaders of influenza in that they excrete the virus in higher concentrations and for longer than adults. Compliance with hygiene measures can be more difficult to maintain and the close proximity in the school setting assists greater efficiency of transmission. For these reasons the scientific advice is that in the event of a significant outbreak schools should close, to protect the children and also to reduce transmission in the wider community. Modelling has suggested that this intervention would help to flatten the peak of an outbreak and therefore reduce the acute demand for healthcare. Even if schools are not closed, it is likely that under these circumstances parents would withdraw their children. Uncertainties remain, however, about when to re-open schools as there is concern that doing so might spark new outbreaks. Whether the shutting of schools will realize the benefits that modellers have predicted remains to be seen. Keeping children apart for substantial periods

R. Puleston

out of school will be challenging and therefore the reductions in infections expected may not be realized.

School closure will have an impact on educational outcomes for children. If they are shut for substantial periods of time, unless steps are taken to enable some continued teaching, children could be disadvantaged. This will be particularly the case for those due to be sitting public examinations. The logistics of accomplishing this while not exposing children and teachers to infection risk will be difficult to achieve.

11.6 Health and Social Care Capacity

During an influenza pandemic the services likely to come under the most pressure are health and social services, and initial planning for pandemic influenza quite rightly concentrates heavily on the response of the healthcare services to ensure patients can be cared for. National guidance focuses on the strategic aspects of responding to a pandemic, giving direction that is then translated at sub-national or regional level for operationalization at the local level – where patients are actually seen. Although some generic decisions can be made – such as to keep influenza patients separate from non-influenza patients – the details of how to do this (e.g. which wards, which part of a hospital, etc.) need to be discussed at the hospital in question, while an overarching body responsible for a region will need to ensure that there is consistency of action between neighbouring hospitals.

Healthcare services are likely to be affected at an early stage in the outbreak and remain under sustained pressure until the end of the outbreak and into the recovery period. Dependent on the severity of the outbreak, demand for health and social care support is likely to rise steeply at the same time as organizations are facing rises in staff absenteeism due to sickness or caring responsibilities. It is probable that at some point during the local epidemic the capacity of these services to respond will be exceeded. Difficult decisions will have to then be taken as to the allocation of these scarce health and social care assets.

Primary and secondary healthcare and social support agencies will have to act at an early stage to prioritize which services to maintain and which to scale back or curtail completely. The implication is that, particularly at the peak of the pandemic, it is possible only the most urgent and ill cases (provided there is a realistic chance of recovery) will be prioritized to access secondary-level healthcare especially intensive care/therapy (where available). Additionally, only the neediest will be provided with direct social support.

Authorities will need to help the remainder of the population to support themselves through the crisis or through access to basic healthcare. Natural and voluntary community support networks will be particularly important for helping the vulnerable through the episode.

Patients will be upset and anxious as routine healthcare appointments become unavailable during the pandemic and it becomes harder to see their doctor as readily as normal. Patients will also be faced with needing to accept that they cannot be admitted to hospital for a complaint that in non-pandemic times would have warranted admission; instead, due to bed shortages during a pandemic, they will have to be cared for at home or using community services.

Existing poor health status

The impact of an influenza pandemic on countries already ravaged by war, poverty and/or other major infectious disease problems (in particular HIV) is likely to be greater than on those not compromised by such difficulties. War, poverty and political breakdown will make it much more difficult for those countries affected to prepare in advance for a major infectious disease outbreak.

Personal protective equipment

The WHO together with individual states' advisory and regulatory bodies has issued guidance on the use of personal protective equipment by certain key staff in a pandemic. Much of this is based on sound reasoning rather than hard evidence. However, it is as yet unclear how successful these measures will be during the crisis, as contemporary real-world usage over a prolonged period has not been experienced in a pandemic situation. Additionally the transmission of the virus is not fully understood and therefore the effectiveness of such equipment is not completely clear (Chapter 5). Given that potentially at-risk workers will need to use the equipment for the duration of each wave which may be as long 15 weeks, compliance with use and availability of supplies may become a problem. Moreover, differences in approaches adopted between and within countries have the potential to cause confusion and divisiveness within the population at large and in specific occupational groups. For example, one European country has procured face masks sufficient for the whole population whereas others have not. Some are advising the use of high-filtration masks for certain exposures while others are advocating that a lower level of protection will be adequate.

Communications and trust

Authorities will need to use effective and reliable communications in order to maintain leadership during an influenza pandemic. In the lead up to and throughout the event, the population will demand information that it can trust. Experience of previous emergencies has demonstrated how important the public's trust in the authorities is and how easily that can be eroded. The financial crisis of 2007–2009 has recently demonstrated how, despite repeated assurances from the regulatory bodies, the population did not trust what they were being told, which in a number of cases led to 'runs' on individual banks. During a pandemic, how will the public respond when seeking reassurance on matters for which there will be much less certainty? Many of the questions they are likely to be ask will have no clear answers. Traditional scepticism around official sources will have to be countered by repeated, consistent and dependable communications. It will be vital that people in positions of authority are transparent and unambiguous in their messages with the public and essential service workforces while minimizing the risks of inducing panic. This will include frankly acknowledging when the state of knowledge is unclear. Tailoring the modes of delivery and language to appropriate groups will be necessary to ensure effective delivery and reach. Balancing all of these needs will be complex (Chapter 13).

R. Puleston

11.7 Conclusions

An influenza pandemic is complex and difficult to plan for because the range of possible impacts is so vast. It may be that the next will be minor and have only marginal effects, or it could be severe with extensive consequences to the social and economic fabric of the world. What is clear is that by careful and effective planning these effects can be mitigated at least in part. However, achieving this without engendering excessive concern, while maintaining sufficient engagement to obtain the resources needed, is complex and will require continued effort by relevant stakeholders if attention is not to be diverted by other competing priorities. Ultimately, an influenza pandemic cannot be tidily packaged as a purely health problem, solvable by a health service-driven solution. Instead, although health remains at the heart of the problem, pandemic influenza is a whole-of-society phenomenon, which demands a whole-of-society response.

11.8 Summary Points

- Pandemic preparedness needs to consider a whole-of-society response because all sectors will be affected over an extended period of time.
- Most businesses are likely to face disruptions to supplies, reduced staffing and reduced demand. Conversely, some business such as food delivery to the home may face an increase in demand.
- While there has been no recent global event of the magnitude anticipated for a future pandemic, there are useful lessons to learn from SARS, Hurricane Katrina, 9/11 and the Indian Ocean tsunami.
- A future influenza pandemic may reduce GDP by up to 5%. The impact will be felt partially through direct effects (e.g. economic losses caused by premature deaths) but also through the consequences of altered patterns of human behaviour.
- Workplace absenteeism will be considerable in a future pandemic, driven by: direct sickness due to influenza and its complications; third-party sickness absence to care for relatives and friends (especially if there are shortages in healthcare capacity); inability to attend work if schools are closed; and refusal to attend work due to fear of catching influenza in the workplace (this may be more common among health and social care workers and teachers).

Further Reading

Gale, J. (2008) *Flu Pandemic May Cost World Economy Up to $3 Trillion (Update3)*. http://www.bloomberg.com/apps/news?pid=20601082&sid=ashmCPWATNwU&refer=canada (accessed May 2009).

Garrett, T.A. (2008) Pandemic economics: the 1918 influenza and its modern-day implications. *Federal Reserve Bank of St Louis Review* 90, 75–93.

Keogh-Brown, M.R. and, Smith R.D. (2008) The economic impact of SARS: how does the reality match the predictions? *Health Policy* 88, 110–120.

Lim, W.S. (2007) Pandemic flu: clinical management of patients with an influenza-like illness during an influenza pandemic. *Thorax* 62(Suppl. 1), 1–46.

Mills, C.E., Robins, J.M. and Lipsitch, M. (2004) Transmissibility of 1918 pandemic influenza. *Nature* 432, 904–906.

Tolle, R., Nunn, P., Maynard, T. and Baxter, D. (2008) *Pandemic, Potential Insurance Effects.* Lloyds, London.

World Health Organization (2003) SARS: lessons from a new disease. In: *The Impact of SARS.* WHO, Geneva, Switzerland, Chapter 5.

R. Puleston

12 Ethical Issues Related to Pandemic Preparedness and Response

E.M. GADD

- How should ethical issues be dealt with in preparing for, and responding to, pandemic influenza?
- Do health professionals have an unlimited obligation to care for patients regardless of the risk to themselves?
- In what circumstances can countries impose mandatory measures to control people's behaviour?
- How can prioritization decisions be addressed in an ethical way?
- Does each country have to work out the answers themselves?

12.1 Introduction

Ethics concerns how it is right to behave. The potential impact on individuals of decisions concerning pandemic preparedness and response means such decisions always have an ethical dimension. The ethical issues involved are often complex and difficult; such issues will be hard to resolve under the pressure of responding to an influenza pandemic, and therefore need to be addressed in advance as far as possible. In addition, an ethical justification is required to treat people in similar circumstances differently. Advance consideration of ethical issues makes it more likely that, at least at national level (given how widely the circumstances of different countries will vary), people will be treated consistently. Consideration of ethical issues should therefore be an integral part of pandemic planning, rather than a separate or side issue.

In complex situations, particularly where resources are limited, there is seldom a single 'right' answer or a solution that could be considered ethically perfect. However, there may be several ethically appropriate or ethically acceptable solutions between which a decision maker can choose. The challenge is to ensure that ethically inappropriate solutions are excluded from consideration.

The ethical issues raised by an influenza pandemic range from wide questions of global justice to medical treatment of individuals. This chapter outlines issues from a health perspective and some of the approaches that countries and international organizations, such as the World Health Organization (WHO), have taken to address them.

12.2 Ethics as an Integral Part of Pandemic Preparedness and Response

As every aspect of pandemic preparedness and response has an ethical dimension, this chapter is not a full account of all the ethical issues that need consideration. Other health issues include, for example, questions concerning management of people detained by the State, whether in prison or on mental health grounds (given that previous pandemics suggest infection rates will be higher in closed institutions), and finding an appropriate balance between the need for medical safeguards in death and cremation certification and the needs of the living for doctors. As ethics concerns how we should behave to others, ethical issues are not confined to the health sector but are also raised by questions concerning, for example, the availability of food and fuel or access to services such as banking or the courts.

Advance preparation is key to an effective response to a pandemic. This raises ethical issues, as countries vary greatly in the resources they can devote to preparation, both in planning terms and in material terms (such as developing a stockpile of antiviral medication). Some developing countries, for example, faced with overwhelming current healthcare needs that cannot be met, have to decide whether it is right to divert any of their limited resources to the task of pandemic planning. In so doing, the potential harms to their population today caused by such diversion must be weighed against the potential future benefits to their population at some unknowable (as the onset of a pandemic cannot be predicted) future date.

12.3 Global Issues and the Role of the World Health Organization

Pandemics respect neither national borders nor the legal status of individuals. For practical purposes, it is reasonable to assume that a pandemic will affect all nations at some point. The shared humanity of individuals globally gives rise to ethical concerns about the inequities between their situations and to an ethical duty to attempt to ameliorate such inequity. At global level, this is often expressed as the principle of solidarity. The ethical duty has been codified into a legal duty of international cooperation and assistance between States expressed in many international human rights instruments, such as the United Nations International Covenant on Economic, Social and Cultural Rights (1966). Article 12 of that Covenant particularly draws attention to that obligation in the context of the prevention, treatment and control of epidemic diseases. Financial aid is not the only form of assistance, for example, sharing of scientific and technological expertise is also important. The WHO is the United Nations body responsible for health and has therefore been responsible for coordinating global pandemic preparedness work.

WHO has recognized the importance of ethical issues in preparedness planning and has produced a series of discussion papers on key issues. These were subject to a consultation with WHO's 193 Member States, after which guidance was produced on ethical considerations in developing a public health response to pandemic influenza.

As well as their legal duties, all States also have reasons of national interest to cooperate. Effective global surveillance offers the opportunity to attempt to control the pandemic at source, and even if this is unsuccessful, provides all States with the maximum possible degree of warning of an imminent pandemic. Achieving such a level of surveillance means that assistance needs to be provided to some States that would not otherwise be able to achieve this goal. Furthermore, timely and effective sharing of scientific information, for example through the sharing of virus and other specimens, has the potential to enhance preparedness and response at global level.

National self-protection is a State's first obligation, and during a pandemic (particularly if it is severe) there will be limits to the international assistance that States can offer. It is ethically important that what is available is used to best effect, and again this requires advance discussion and planning, incorporating the flexibility to respond according to the characteristics of the pandemic.

The legal status of individuals is often relevant to access to national healthcare systems. The position of asylum seekers, refugees and displaced people during a pandemic therefore needs consideration. Many countries have reciprocal health agreements regarding the medical treatment of their citizens who become ill on the territory of the other country, but these are not universal. The treatment of citizens of States with whom no agreement exists therefore also needs thought. As well as the ethical issues, the sheer practicality of healthcare staff making enquiries about a person's legal status under the pressures of a pandemic has to be considered.

'Health tourism' during a pandemic, in which people attempt to travel from a country thought to be ill-resourced or ill-prepared to another seen as being in a better situation, could present difficulties. Where countries share borders such travel may be relatively easy. The ethical dimensions of such a practice are quite complex, involving consideration of the position of others in both the original and receiving countries. It may be preferable to minimize the risks of the practice developing, both for ethical reasons and because of the potential disruption to pandemic response that might occur from such a practice if widespread. WHO has highlighted the need to try to avoid disparities of care across borders, and this is another reason for neighbouring countries to cooperate in planning for a pandemic.

The pressures involved in planning for, and responding to, a pandemic mean that the need to plan for the recovery phase can be overlooked. International cooperation and assistance will again be important. While the full range of difficulties that countries may face in the recovery phase cannot be discussed here, the existing inequities between countries in terms of healthcare staff and services can be highlighted. Where few staff are available even in normal times, the loss of a critical number of these during a pandemic may produce an ongoing crisis in healthcare provision. The need for assistance both in terms of shoring up available provision and in training new staff may be profound.

12.4 Voluntary and Mandatory Non-medical Measures

Given the different resources available to them, countries will vary in the extent to which they can use medical measures such as antiviral medication or hospital care to respond to a pandemic. The use of some non-medical measures, such as border controls and entry or exit screening (even if largely ineffective – see Chapter 7), also has resource consequences. However, measures such as isolation or quarantine may be relevant to a wide range of countries, although the potential to enforce such measures will vary widely.

The right to associate freely with others and not to be deprived of liberty without just cause are recognized in international human rights instruments at both the global and regional level (e.g. in the European Convention for the Protection of Human Rights and Fundamental Freedoms (ECHR)). These support the ethical principle of self-determination, or autonomy. However, the international legal instruments do recognize that these rights can legitimately be limited in certain circumstances, including the need to protect public health.

However, not all restrictions are legitimate. The Siracusa Principles, as noted in WHO's guidance on ethical considerations referred to above, are widely accepted as a standard for assessment of the legitimacy of a restriction on human rights. These are that the restriction is: in accordance with law; based on a legitimate objective; the least restrictive and intrusive means available; and not arbitrary, unreasonable or discriminatory.

What does this mean in practice? In the first place, there must be a reasonable belief that the proposed measure would be effective. Chapter 7 shows that modelling estimates that even massive restrictions on air travel would be unlikely to have a significant effect on the impact of a pandemic in the UK – which leads to the conclusion that it would be unreasonable for the State to impose such a measure. It is ethically less problematic to encourage people to cooperate voluntarily with a measure than to impose it, although if a measure cannot work in any circumstances there are no grounds for seeking voluntary cooperation. For a measure to be the least restrictive and intrusive means available, there must be reasonable grounds to believe that voluntary measures will not be effective and mandatory measures will.

If a voluntary measure would not be effective, consideration must be given to the feasibility of enforcing a mandatory measure. For example, even in an influenza pandemic with a relatively low clinical attack rate of 25%, how feasible would it be to enforce home isolation? How could that be monitored? Large-scale enforcement problems give rise to concerns as to whether the measure can be effected in a way that is not arbitrary. Furthermore, the benefits that can be achieved need to be proportionate to the burdens placed on individuals by a mandatory measure. By imposing and enforcing a measure for collective benefit, the State also has an ethical obligation to minimize the harm that it causes to the relevant individuals. So, for example, if a person were to be confined at home, attention needs to be given to the provision of food, medical care and other necessities of life to that person.

It is important to distinguish between measures that individuals choose for themselves, such as not to go to a mass gathering or other place that the person anticipates being crowded in order to avoid infection, and measures imposed by the State. Imposed measures that limit the freedom of individuals require rigorous justification, balancing the potential collective benefits to society against the rights of individuals. This is a difficult test; it is much less ethically problematic to encourage people to cooperate voluntarily with measures that are likely to benefit society (such as isolation at home when ill with influenza) than to legally impose such measures.

Where voluntary measures are used, providing individuals with information that explains the reasons why the measure is encouraged demonstrates respect for people and supports the right to self-determination. There may be situations where the scientific evidence indicates that at population level a measure (such as avoiding mass gatherings) would make no, or minimal, difference to the impact of the pandemic.

E.M. Gadd

In such circumstances, it would be ethically appropriate to provide what information is available on the potential risks at individual level, and allow people to make their own choices on how to behave as a result.

Considering the ethical dimensions of a potential measure requires thinking about the potential impact on all those who may be affected by a decision. School closures are a good example. Obvious issues are harms through loss of educational opportunities and association with friends for the children, coupled with potential benefits in terms of reduced rates of infection for the children and (probably) in society more widely. But if schools are closed, childcare will be needed. This may present few problems in societies in which hardly any women work outside the home, but for societies in which it is common for both parents to work the impact may be far more significant. In such societies, sectors that employ a high proportion of working parents (particularly women), which will already be experiencing absenteeism through the direct health impact of a pandemic, may then be placed under an additional burden as parents face the conflict between their domestic and work responsibilities, and this in turn may give rise to societal harms.

The extensive potential impact of school closures in some societies means that is impossible to judge the best course of action until the exact characteristics of a pandemic virus are known; what would be appropriate may differ depending on the clinical attack rate, mortality rate and differing vulnerabilities of sub-sections of the population associated with the virus. If school closures are a potential option in such countries, in order to minimize harms, society (and particularly sectors that may be disproportionately affected) needs to be aware of this well in advance so that individuals and organizations can incorporate it in their plans.

12.5 Health Professionals' Duty of Care

An influenza pandemic will place severe demands on healthcare services, and health professionals will be key to an effective response. But they will also face conflicting obligations, for example to family members, and particularly if the pandemic virus is associated with a high mortality rate, may be placed at higher risk as a result of their professional duties.

The extent of health professionals' duty of care has been debated. Sources of the duty include ethical and professional obligations as well as contractual and other legal duties. This section focuses on the situation in developed countries, rather than situations in which lack of health professionals is always a major problem.

Ethical obligations may arise from the specialized knowledge possessed by health professionals, particularly if their training has been funded by the State. Professionals may also feel an ethical obligation to work from solidarity with their colleagues, recognizing the burden that their absence places on others. Professional obligations derive from professional codes of conduct that require giving care, particularly in emergency situations. However, there is no universal agreement on the extent of the obligation, although there seems to be broad agreement (as expressed in WHO's guidance on ethical considerations referred to above) that the extent is not unlimited. In addition, in some cases, for example due to a personal medical condition, caring for someone with an infectious disease might place a particular health professional at unusually high risk, and this also needs ethical consideration.

Historically, the professional response to serious infectious disease has been mixed. While there are examples of great heroism, there are also examples where doctors are reported to have fled the area. The recent experience of severe acute respiratory syndrome (SARS) provides an opportunity to examine this issue in a modern context. An important factor to recall with SARS, which will not be relevant to pandemic influenza, is that for some time the actual cause of SARS was not known. In addition, SARS in the developed world was largely confined to healthcare institutions. The risk of infection outside such institutions was negligible. In contrast, during an influenza pandemic, levels of infection in the community will be significant; a health professional may be exposed to infection travelling between work and home, while carrying out domestic tasks such as shopping or in the course of family life. Not working is therefore no guarantee of avoiding infection.

During SARS, the majority of health professionals demonstrated high commitment to care (as a result of which some died), but this was not universal. The SARS experience suggests that keeping staff well informed of developments, the provision of personal protective equipment, and a non-punitive approach to those who felt unable to undertake direct care, may contribute to an effective response to pandemic influenza.

Attempts have been made to study health professionals' attitudes to working during an influenza pandemic. Studies of health workers in Europe and the USA suggest that a significant number thought that they might not report for work, although clinical staff appeared significantly more likely to intend to work than non-clinical or support staff. Perception of the importance of one's role in responding to a pandemic appeared to be a significant factor. Fear of infection of oneself or family was raised as a reason for not working, but as noted above it may not be realistic to expect to avoid infection by avoiding work.

The need for information and for reciprocity – in terms of provision of protective equipment and expression of appreciation of the potential burdens staff may assume – has also been highlighted. In addition, staff may fear that the pressures of a pandemic may mean that they will be unable to deliver their normal standard of care, or that they may need to work in unfamiliar areas or take on new roles, and that this might have medico-legal consequences. Inappropriate care during a pandemic would always be regrettable, but (depending on the particular circumstances) it may not be appropriate to consider it ethically blameworthy. If health professionals deliver the best care they can during a pandemic, there is an ethical obligation to minimize the professional or employment consequences of so doing.

Involving health professionals – and indeed other staff – at an early stage in pandemic planning is important to gain commitment to cooperation in pandemic response. Such discussions should aim to clarify expectations concerning the duties of health professionals and to provide information, so far as it is known, about the potential risks of pandemic influenza and delivering care and about the measures available to support staff (including personal protective equipment, access to medicines or vaccines, etc.). Early discussions also provide the opportunity to address individual issues, such as personal health needs or childcare, which could impact on the person's ability to deliver care. A person may be able to contribute to the pandemic response in other ways (e.g. staffing an advisory telephone helpline).

The ethical obligations of health professionals to patients are widely recognized; in pandemic preparedness and response it is also necessary for society, and in particular for those directing the preparedness and response phases, to remember the ethical obligations to those, including but not limited to health professionals, on whom the burden of response may fall particularly heavily.

12.6 Prioritization and Access to Healthcare

Questions of prioritization for access to healthcare are not new, although an influenza pandemic is likely to present them in a more severe form. Many different approaches to healthcare prioritization and rationing have been proposed, but there is no general agreement on the best method – although it is clear that some approaches are less ethically acceptable than others. How a country approaches these issues during a pandemic will be dependent on the resources available to it, in terms of both the healthcare system and its staff and specific interventions such as antiviral medication and vaccines.

The potential impact of prioritization on individuals means that it is ethically highly desirable to involve society to the greatest extent possible in the process for deciding the approach and criteria to be used. Wide social understanding and acceptance of the chosen approach is also likely to facilitate the management of the pandemic.

In terms of general approach, when considering issues at a population level, the principle that one should do 'the greatest good for the greatest number' is often proposed. This principle of utility is not as straightforward as it seems, and has a practical impact on the choice of prioritization criteria. Ideas of what constitutes the 'greatest good' may vary – options include: minimizing the clinical attack rate so that fewer people are affected; minimizing deaths; maximizing health benefits by saving most life-years (resulting in lowered priority for older people); and taking a wider view and aiming to minimize the impact of a pandemic on society (which leads to considerations of individuals' social roles and their impact on society). Some type of utility consideration will form part of any prioritization approach, but the form this takes may vary in different circumstances, such as the use of pre-pandemic vaccine or access to intensive care.

However, utility considerations fail to address significant ethical concerns. For example, if there are five items of a limited resource and many people who could benefit equally from it, the maximum number of people who can receive the resource is five. But most people would think there is an ethical difference between choosing the five by lottery or the person responsible for the resource choosing five friends over the other potential beneficiaries. This reflects an underlying concern with fairness, or equity, which concerns giving equal weight to equal claims.

In normal circumstances, equity considerations generally support giving priority to the worst off – in a casualty department, the sickest people are treated first, and those who will not be harmed by having to wait do so. Such considerations are also relevant in a pandemic, for example, one could consider prioritizing groups of people who may be at higher risk of death if infected to receive vaccine. However, considerations of equity may conflict with utility and a difficult balance may have to be found. For example, one very sick person with multiple underlying medical conditions might need to occupy a ventilator bed for several weeks to stand a chance of recovery. In that time, many other people who needed the ventilator for only a short period in order to make a full recovery could die.

These potential conflicts need to be widely debated in advance in order to reach agreement on the limitations to treatment that can be offered. Such limitations may vary depending on the pressures on the limited resource and other options available; it is ethically desirable that limitations are applied only to the extent necessary, so the application of a particular level of limitation needs to be kept under regular review. However, even with the strictest restrictions based on medical criteria in force, particularly in a severe pandemic, there may be more people with equal claims to, for example, an intensive-care bed than there are beds available. Very hard choices will need to be made – on equity grounds, these need to be made fairly but also in a way that is practical in the situation. 'First come first served' approaches are difficult to operationalize fairly; how do you assess 'first'? The first person notified to the intensive-care consultant after the bed becomes available? What if a person tried to call the consultant, who was otherwise occupied, and before the person called back another notification was made? A lottery between patients with an equal claim to the bed may be a more practical (and fair) answer, but thought is needed as to how this would be implemented in practice.

The use of age in prioritization is very controversial. An equity-based argument that has been much discussed is the 'fair innings' approach. This suggests that a young person may have a stronger claim to life-saving treatment than an older person who has already had a 'fair innings'. However, this makes age the defining characteristic of an individual and ignores other characteristics that might be ethically relevant. Furthermore, defining the cut-off for a 'fair innings' in the real world is always going to be fraught with difficulty. Age may sometimes be relevant in prioritization, for example, if there is scientific evidence that the ageing of the body means statistically that persons of a certain age are less likely to respond to certain forms of treatment, on utility grounds this may be relevant to considering potential benefits from treatment. But it is not based on the concept of a 'fair innings' and needs to be tempered by consideration of the individual (some 70-year-olds are fitter than some 30-year-olds), so population-level data should not be applied blindly.

There are some criteria that can never be appropriate for use in prioritization, such as gender, religion, sexual orientation, political affiliation or socio-economic status. The prohibition of unjustified discrimination is emphasized in legal human rights documents at global and regional level (such as the ECHR) and this applies in a pandemic as at other times.

During a pandemic, people will still have road accidents, heart attacks, strokes, develop cancers and give birth. Those affected also have ethical claims to care, and this needs to be taken into account in pandemic planning and prioritization criteria for resources that both they and patients with influenza-related illness may need, such as intensive care. Consideration also needs to be given to the potential impact of decreasing preventive care such as childhood immunization during a pandemic, given that potentially severe childhood illnesses such as measles and whooping cough will remain risks.

As noted above, the needs of those who are 'worst off' require consideration on grounds of equity. In developed countries, many disabled, frail and otherwise vulnerable people are dependent on social care, often for many basic activities of daily living such as meals, dressing and bathing. Social care staff will be affected as others in society by a pandemic, and the impact of absenteeism on social services needs careful consideration.

As noted at the start of this section, the importance and effects of prioritization decisions are such that they need to be subject to the widest possible debate during the preparedness planning phase. Protocols need to be developed and discussed on issues such as limitations to care (such as in relation to intensive care) and made publicly available. How these will be reviewed (e.g. to take account of emerging information on the pandemic virus) needs to be made clear. It is important to ensure that all members of society can contribute to the debate (not everyone uses the Internet), and so making information available in community languages, large print and other formats and accessible to groups such as the homeless or travellers is important. The use of transparently developed, publicly available criteria will be important in assuring people that the principles agreed are being applied fairly in individual cases during the pandemic itself, and this will assist in maintaining public trust in the management of the pandemic.

12.7 National Approaches to Ethical Issues

The importance of addressing the ethical dimension of managing an influenza pandemic has been recognized worldwide. This has been achieved in different ways, and informed by academic contributions. Of these, *Stand on Guard for Thee*, a report of the University of Toronto Joint Centre for Bioethics, is notable. This built on the work of the Centre after the Canadian SARS outbreak and proposes a series of ethical and procedural values to inform pandemic planning.

Some countries have an existing national ethics committee that has looked at pandemic influenza as well as other problems. Examples include the Swiss National Advisory Committee on Biomedical Ethics, whose contribution was integrated into the Swiss Influenza Pandemic Plan. The New Zealand National Ethics Advisory Committee has produced detailed, separate guidance on ethical values for a pandemic. Its guidance also provides a range of hypothetical scenarios from an influenza pandemic that are used to illustrate the practical implementation of the ethical values proposed.

The UK does not have a general national ethics committee, but subject-specific national committees. The Government therefore set up the Committee on Ethical Aspects of Pandemic Influenza. This produced an ethical framework for policy and planning that was accepted by the Government and now forms part of the pandemic response. The Committee was also consulted on planning preparedness guidance in draft on a range of issues.

Approaches based on setting out frameworks of principles or values recognize the impracticality of an ethics committee providing a precise answer on every ethical question that may arise in pandemic management. The principles may often be in tension, as noted with issues of equity and utility above, and how this tension is to be balanced will depend on the exact circumstances under consideration. Furthermore, as scientific information changes (e.g. concerning the characteristics of a new pandemic virus) this may impact on ethical decisions, and plans need to be flexible enough to take this into account. Frameworks of values or principles can act as a decision support tool, by encouraging people to consider systematically the different ethical dimensions of a problem. Those involved in the management of a pandemic are expected to be aware of the framework and to use it to inform their daily decision making where this is not covered by specific protocols (e.g. concerning limitations of care in certain circumstances).

As one might hope, there is considerable commonality between the approaches to setting out values or principles. For example, both the UK and New Zealand frameworks specify minimizing harm, and call for respect, fairness and reciprocity and (expressed in different words) working together, flexibility and procedural principles related to good decision making. The UK also has a principle of keeping things in proportion, and New Zealand a value of responsibleness, but it seems probable that if these slightly different frameworks were applied to the same situation the outcome would be very similar.

However, a framework is not a calculator – one cannot hypothetically feed an issue in at one end and expect a precise answer to simply emerge. Judgement is always required about the weight to be given to a particular principle in a specific situation; or with a broad principle such as minimizing harm, about which harms are particularly important. That is why the element of the frameworks dealing with good decision making is particularly important, as this aims to ensure that those difficult judgements are made in the most ethically appropriate manner.

Ultimately, all of those responsible for planning and responding to pandemic influenza need to be aware of the ethical dimensions of their work, and to ensure that ethical issues are appropriately addressed in the decisions they take. As this chapter has illustrated, the complexity of the issues is such that, in terms of ensuring an ethically appropriate response to a pandemic, the benefits of thinking things through in advance of the pandemic cannot be overstated.

12.8   Summary Points

- All decisions that affect people have an ethical dimension, so ethical issues need to be integrated into the preparations for, and response to, pandemic influenza.
- Health professionals have a strong duty to care, but it is not unlimited. Willingness to care is enhanced by recognizing reciprocal obligations to health professionals (e.g. to consult them, provide protective equipment and keep them informed of developments).
- Mandatory measures can only be imposed if voluntary measures would be ineffective, and must meet certain legal criteria if they are to be legitimate.
- Criteria for prioritization decisions need to be subject to wide public discussion. Such criteria will involve a balance between ethical principles of utility and fairness and must avoid unjustified discrimination.
- International legal agreements mean countries have a duty to work together, and WHO has produced guidance on ethical considerations related to a pandemic. Countries take this into account in producing national guidance on ethical issues, such as frameworks of values or principles to inform the national response.

Further Reading

Cabinet Office and Department of Health (2007) *Responding to pandemic influenza: The ethical framework for policy and planning.* http://www.dh.gov.uk/en/Publicationsandsta tistics/Publications/PublicationsPolicyAndGuidance/DH_080751 (accessed May 2009).

New Zealand National Ethics Advisory Committee (2007) *Getting Through Together: Ethical values for a pandemic*. http://www.neac.health.govt.nz/moh.nsf/pagescm/1090/$File/ getting-through-together-jul07.pdf (accessed May 2009).

University of Toronto Joint Centre for Bioethics (2005) *Stand on Guard for Thee. Ethical considerations in preparedness planning for pandemic influenza*. A report of the University of Toronto Joint Centre for Bioethics Pandemic Influenza Working Group. http://www. jointcentreforbioethics.ca/publications/documents/stand_on_guard.pdf (accessed May 2009).

World Health Organization (2007) *Ethical considerations in developing a public health response to pandemic influenza*. http://www.who.int/csr/resources/publications/WHO_ CDS_EPR_GIP_2007_2c.pdf (accessed May 2009).

World Health Organization (2008) *Addressing ethical issues in pandemic influenza planning: discussion papers*. http://www.who.int/csr/resources/publications/cds_flu_ethics_5web. pdf (accessed May 2009).

13 Communication with the Public

E. COLLINS

- Why communicate with the public about pandemic influenza?
- Whose responsibility is it to talk to the public and when?
- What is the best way to communicate with the public?
- What messages should be communicated during an influenza pandemic?
- Why is it important to communicate internally?

13.1 Introduction

There are a number of features of pandemic influenza that are almost inevitable and guarantee that a future pandemic will cause of a great deal of concern among the public. Something on a worldwide scale that has the ability to disrupt normal life in this way requires careful communications handling over a long period of time to ensure the public are well prepared and that key messages about how they can protect themselves and their families, and how they should go about their daily lives, are well understood.

During a pandemic, governments, public health authorities and the third sector (e.g. charities, non-governmental organizations and voluntary organizations) will have responsibility for communicating with the public; this chapter is aimed primarily at those organizations. However it should be noted that almost all private sector (business) organizations, while having less in the way of a public health responsibility, will be inextricably caught up in the crisis because of their interface with consumers (the public at large) and the need to manage individual businesses through the crisis (see Chapters 6 and 11).

Some emergency situations, for example a bio-terrorist release of an infectious disease, would lead to a very immediate demand for information from the public and media. However, in communication terms, a pandemic is a more slowly emerging scenario and would result in a period of time (1 or 2 weeks) during the early phases when public messages can be reiterated on a regular basis and through a variety of means, to ensure the public are more prepared when cases start to occur in their locality.

Most organizations will have a communications professional employed to liaise with the public and media as well as communicate internally with staff. This role may exist as part of a press office, a public relations team or a wider communications team. All material destined for the public domain and for the purpose of public education and communication will usually go through the communications team so that they can ensure consistency in public materials and that these are appropriately pitched (in terms of language and complexity) for their intended audience, and finally

---

©CAB International 2010. *Introduction to Pandemic Influenza*
(eds J.S. Nguyen-Van-Tam and C. Sellwood)

Focus Box 13.1. Features of pandemic influenza that will generate public concern.

- Between 25 and 40% of people may become ill with symptoms, so, even if mild, a pandemic will affect most households.
- There will be increased deaths, including some in children and young adults.
- It is almost certain that international and domestic travel will decline spontaneously and travel disruptions may occur due to staff shortages.
- Even though it may not be an effective public health strategy, certain large gatherings may be voluntarily cancelled (e.g. sporting fixtures and concerts).
- Healthcare demand is likely to exceed capacity at the peak of the pandemic; people will not like this.
- In countries that have stockpiles of antiviral drugs, there will be active encouragement to come forward for treatment early.
- There may be short-term disruption to essential supplies and commodities, such as food, fuel and power.
- Schools may close for a period.

that they are shared with other stakeholder organizations. It is crucial to become familiar with the communications team and its protocols, at the earliest possible opportunity.

Ahead of a pandemic it is important to develop a communications strategy. This should set out the messages that will be shared, the channels that will be used and who is responsible for this. It is important to identify key spokespeople in advance and to ensure they have received media training so that they are confident and comfortable when speaking to broadcast and print journalists. It is also recommended that the strategy is tested regularly using exercise scenarios and updated regularly in the light of new information, changes within the organization or other developments that might impact its effectiveness.

13.2 Getting the Message Across

Public communication before and during a crisis such as an influenza pandemic is crucial for a number of reasons:

- It will educate people about pandemic influenza and how it differs from avian or normal seasonal influenza.
- It will provide people with the relevant health information they need about influenza and what to do if they have symptoms.
- It will encourage the public to follow advice and behave in a way that protects the wider community, for example following hygiene measures and disposing of used tissues in the correct way.
- It will ensure that the public know how to go about their daily lives during a pandemic and what they are being advised to do.
- It will ensure that the public know how the pandemic is being handled by all the organizations involved and what plans are in place to protect them.

13.3 World Health Organization Principles for Outbreak Communication

The World Health Organization (WHO) has developed five key principles of outbreak communication guidelines for use during outbreaks of infectious disease (Table 13.1).

These are simple and obvious principles, but ensuring they are followed can make the difference between a successful communications campaign and an ineffective campaign full of angst, mixed messages and rumour.

Consistency of messages

Before any information is communicated to the public, staff or media it is important to decide upon the key messages; these are likely to differ depending on the stage of the pandemic. These key messages should then be used in any press releases, public information such as leaflets and factsheets, or in any media interviews. It is important that messages are consistent with those of the lead organization in your country, which would most probably be the government department responsible for health. If messages are not consistent, then this will lead to confusion among the general public, who will be in receipt of different information, from different organizations, and may not know which piece of information to follow. Messages also need to be consistent at the local level – between multi-agency partners such as health and non-health, local government authorities, police, the voluntary sector and all others involved in responding to the situation.

The importance of language

To ensure that recipients will understand your messages, it is essential to use simple, non-technical language and avoid complex scientific terminology. Being familiar with a subject, or being a specialist in a particular area, makes it easy to take for granted that others will speak the same technical language, however, it is important to go

Table 13.1. The World Health Organization's five key principles of outbreak communication.

Trust	Building, maintaining and restoring trust between the public and the organizations involved in responding to the incident
Announcing early	Providing the most up-to-date information as soon as possible – good news should be shared as soon as it is available, and bad news does not get better if it is held back
Transparency	Giving timely, accurate and full information promptly, and sharing new information proactively
Listening	Understanding the audience's fears and concerns so that information is relevant to them
Planning	Communications planning is essential – in order to be able to respond reactively but also to act proactively as much as possible

E. Collins

> **Focus Box 13.2. Examples of 'jargon' or non-standard language around pandemic influenza.**
>
> - Respiratory hygiene (quite technical).
> - Waves (e.g. people may not realize this means subsequent bouts of the illness in the population).
> - Antivirals ('anti-what?').
> - Pandemic (how does this differ from the more familiar term 'epidemic'?).

back to basics when writing for the public and ensure all information is pitched at a level that will be understood by everyone. If language is simple and unambiguous then this means there is more chance of the public following advice and being reassured by it, rather than being confused by it.

Information should be laid out clearly, and should use short sentences and good punctuation so that any instructions are simple, unambiguous and easy to understand. It is important to think very carefully about the audience; for example, about what their level of knowledge is, their literacy levels and also what will be important to them. Messages can then be tailored so they are relevant to their needs, which in turn will mean that people are more likely to take information on board, remember it and act upon it when the time comes.

13.4 Media Communications

Research in the UK has shown that during any kind of emergency, the two main formal sources people go to for information are the television and radio. This does not imply that other sources such as newspapers, the Internet or websites should be ignored – if anything, it is important to have a communications strategy that encompasses a number of different channels so that different audiences can be reached. Information is more likely to be remembered if it has been received through a number of different sources, for example, read in a paper, seen on a billboard advertisement and then watched on the television.

With 24-hour news and an ever-increasing number of news outlets, the demand for information from the media during a pandemic will be intense. This demand will be placed on all organizations that have a role in protecting the public and ensuring public services run, and will also extend to organizations whose outputs are affected through staff shortages arising as a result of a pandemic. Because a pandemic is projected to last for about 4 months and may involve more than one wave of disease in the population, it is important that any communications department/team is well equipped to respond to this and has the necessary strategy and staffing to cover this period. It might be wise for some communications departments to seek help and secure agreements from colleagues elsewhere in the organization or externally, as 'back-ups' ahead of a pandemic, and ensure the necessary training has been given and these colleagues know what their role will involve should they be called upon. Each organization will have its own media handling protocols; however, in a time of emergency it is strongly recommended to be as open as possible with the media and to exploit its power to help inform the public about influenza and what people can do to protect themselves and others.

The media will need new angles for their stories each day and it is therefore recommended that figures on the progress of the pandemic are released at the same time each day so media become accustomed to routine availability. Again this is likely to be carried out by the lead government department. Even if your organization has nothing new to say, then make the media aware of this when they call and let them know when you are likely to have new information for them.

Prior to a pandemic it is important to build up a list of journalists or media contacts who you can call on in a pandemic to help communicate the information. A relationship can be built up with these journalists and they can be informed about your organization and its role, so all of this background is well understood prior to the crisis beginning. Organizations like the UK British Broadcasting Corporation (BBC) are a good place to start as they have a public service remit and run work streams such as 'connecting in a crisis', where they work with organizations ahead of a crisis, to enable them to deliver good public information when the need arises.

It is crucial to involve both national and local media – the latter is more trusted by the general public, and so is an essential part of the communications process.

Another information source that is especially relevant and well-trusted is a more informal source: word of mouth. This is the main conduit via which most people receive new information, and it is (depending on the source) often a very trusted channel. Research in the UK has indicated that these informal sources (such as family members or health service/public sector employees) will be trusted far more than 'official' governmental sources. Of course, it is impossible to control this information source – but it is very important to keep in mind that employees and stakeholders at your organization are often sought-after and trusted information sources for their friends and family in a crisis like this one. It will be essential to keep staff and stakeholders very well informed so that the 'word-of-mouth' information sources coming out of your organization are as accurate as the more formal information sources. A later section of this chapter discusses the specific issue of communicating with staff.

Finally, the recent rapid rise of 'citizen journalism' through Internet personal web logs (or 'blogs') provides an unrivalled and almost unregulated mechanism for informal communication, including ill-informed rumour mongering and conspiracy theorizing. Mainstream print and broadcast channels often include a 'round up of the blogs' and as such potentially give these sites and the information they contain an inappropriate air of credibility. It is important as part of your communications activity to monitor these more informal internet sources, where possible, to see what kind of information is being included in them.

13.5 Spokespeople and Trust

For the purpose of recognition it is important that the public become familiar with the people who are providing them with information and advice. It is therefore recommended that an organization chooses two or three spokespeople, where possible, who can carry out all media interviews. These people should not be too intricately involved in the response itself and should be available at very short notice. A spokesperson does not have to be someone who is your leading expert on the topic itself; however, they do need to be clearly spoken, well presented, a good communicator and, most importantly, well briefed about the topic area. It is particularly important to identify more than one spokesperson due to the extended duration of a pandemic (up to 15 weeks per wave) to ensure there is a degree of resilience in relation to communicating externally, as well as the very real risk that your spokesperson could well get ill themselves during the pandemic.

To ensure the public listen to and follow advice from your organization it is important to build up a trusted reputation ahead of any crisis. This can be done by being as open as possible with the public and media and ensuring that any negative stories are well managed.

Public research in the UK has shown that doctors are the most trusted source of information, with 90% of the population questioned citing doctors as the people they would most trust. Scientists are also well trusted by 72% of the population. With this research in mind it is recommended that, where possible, scientists and doctors within the organization are chosen to speak to the media, rather than non-medical or non-scientific staff. Public trust can vary in scientists depending on how their work is funded, with those funded by the government being less trusted than those funded by a charity or environmental group, for example. The same research also showed that at the bottom end of the scale of trust were politicians and journalists, and that only one in five people will trust information they receive from a government minister. It is therefore crucial that these spokespeople's messages do reinforce the national messages from government or health bodies, to reassure the public.

13.6   A Varied Communications Strategy

An effective communications strategy will include many different forms of communication. This will ensure as many people as possible receive the correct information. Channels other than television and radio can include the use of an official website and recorded information for those phoning the organization. Leaflets and adverts can also be used, if funding will allow, and these plans should tie in with those of the lead government department.

A simple way for the public to access information during a pandemic is through websites, so it is vital that the organization's website is available during a pandemic. It should also be updated regularly, so visitors to the site can access information about the latest advice and any new developments. As demand for information via a website will increase during an emergency like a pandemic, it is recommended that testing is carried out ahead of time to ensure the site can accommodate the increased level of visitors expected. It is also important to ensure the site links through to any related organizations that also provide information on pandemic influenza, so the public have easy access to all the information that is available.

Another important communications conduit is staff members themselves, especially so in health or social care organizations. They are a trusted source of information for their friends and family, and can almost be seen as 'ambassadors' of information in this context. It is essential to get them 'on board' early on in the process and, above all, ensure they are kept fully informed, involved and up to date on events and messages.

13.7   Message Timing and Intensity

It is important prior to a pandemic (i.e. in WHO Pandemic Alert Phases 3 and 4) not to overload the public with information or enter into a 'cry wolf' scenario whereby people do not believe the pandemic will ever happen and therefore stop listening to information. This happened to some degree with the 'Year 2000' computer bug, where significant effort was placed into ensuring electronic goods were able to 'survive' when internal clocks changed from 31 December 1999 (311299) to 1 January 2000 (010100). In the event, there were no major information technology problems linked with the date change and life carried on as before, leaving the public wondering what all the fuss had been about.

During the early stages it will be necessary to familiarize the public with information about how a pandemic differs from avian or seasonal influenza. Research has shown that public understanding of pandemic influenza is limited and the risk is that this can lead to confusion with other types of influenza, about whether vaccines will be available and which groups are more likely to be affected. Messages should also reinforce the need for hand hygiene and the importance of practising hand hygiene to protect yourself and those around you. Campaigns that can be referred to on this issue include the recent Department of Health, England's campaign 'Catch It! Bin It! Kill It!', which reinforces messages about the use of tissues and hygiene when suffering from a cold or flu (Fig. 13.1).

Research among the UK public during 2007 showed that when questioned about their top health threats, 6% spontaneously mentioned avian or bird influenza as a concern, and when actually given a list of threats to choose from, 11% cited avian influenza as a concern. Most people attribute their concerns to what they have read about in newspapers, so this figure may rise at times when there is a lot of coverage of avian and pandemic influenza in the news, and fall when there is less reporting.

When cases are anticipated imminently or have just started occurring in a country, the public will need more information about how to recognize the symptoms of influenza and what to do if they or a family member should become ill. This information may include the benefits of antivirals and how they can obtain these if they need them. Regular updates should also be provided about public service disruption and how this may affect people's daily lives, including the need for school closures and that families should consider making alternative arrangements in advance of such an event.

13.8   Recovery Phase

In the recovery phase after a pandemic it will be important to remind people that services will take some time to return to normal and patience will be required during this period. This is also a good time to thank the public for their cooperation with

E. Collins

(a)

CATCH IT

Germs spread easily. Always carry tissues and use them to catch your cough or sneeze.

BIN IT

Germs can live for several hours on tissues. Dispose of your tissue as soon as possible.

KILL IT

Hands can transfer germs to every surface you touch. Clean your hands as soon as you can.

NHS

(b)

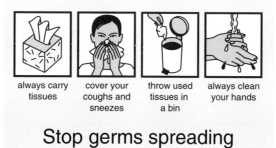

NHS

Coughs and sneezes spread diseases

| always carry tissues | cover your coughs and sneezes | throw used tissues in a bin | always clean your hands |

Stop germs spreading

Fig. 13.1. (a) Catch It! Bin It! Kill It! (illustration by Anthony Burrill) and (b) Coughs and sneezes (Crown Copyright, reproduced under the terms of the Click-Use Licence). (Reproduced with kind permission of the Department of Health, England.)

Focus Box 13.3. Examples of pandemic communication challenges.

- Giving healthy people confidence to continue using mass transportation systems.
- Explaining the purpose of school closures and the importance of avoiding alternative childcare arrangements where children can again mix (e.g. street corner crèches).
- Explaining why seasonal influenza vaccine is of no benefit against pandemic influenza and why pandemic vaccine could not have been made any sooner.
- Explaining a second wave after the first is over.
- Explaining why port-of-entry screening is not likely to be effective.
- Explaining why there will be further pandemic influenza cases when schools re-open.
- In the case of antiviral drugs running out, explaining why this has happened.
- In the case of a pandemic virus that has resistance properties, explaining why one or more stockpiled drugs will not work.
- Explaining why most people who need treatment cannot be seen by a doctor.

This list is not intended to be exhaustive, but to illustrate the range of particularly difficult pandemic-specific communication challenges.

any messages and information for which your organization has been responsible. If there is a decline in activity before a second wave of the pandemic, then all the same messages from before the pandemic can be reinforced, providing these remain appropriate and relevent.

13.9 Local Communications

The communications needs on a local level will be slightly different from those at national level. The pandemic may affect different areas at different times and therefore messages may be needed earlier or later. It is possible that schools in one area of a country will be closed before another or the rates of influenza will be much higher in one area than another, and all these differences will necessitate targeted communications so the public are aware of the localized situation and what they need to do. The public will also require more local information about where they can seek medical help and advice and where they should go for antivirals. Local media and web sites can be used to communicate this kind of information to the target populations.

The makeup of the local population should be taken into account, especially regarding whether different forms of communication or translations into multiple languages may be required. In some countries, several different languages may be spoken by indigenous people, while in others it may be a legal requirement for information to be translated into multiple languages, for example in Canada where both English and French are spoken. Translating information can be further complicated by the existence of different dialects, for example in Kurdish and Punjabi, while some languages, such as Somali, did not exist in written form until the 1970s.

In some Westernized countries, there are differences in the societal organization and networks of recent immigrant groups as opposed to those that are longer

E. Collins

established in a 'foreign' country. Within the UK, for example, it is thought that there are very few people who are genuinely monoglot in a language other than English and/or who do not have an English-speaking family member or friend. Expatriate media services, which many groups establish in their own language, can be a useful tool when communicating with large communities of non-native speakers and it is important to ensure these media outlets are kept informed of key messages.

Harder-to-reach populations in the community should also be considered in any communications strategy, and options should be available to communicate with those who have physical disabilities including sight and hearing disabilities, those with learning and/or mental health difficulties and also those with literacy or information access constraints. AIDS/sexually transmitted disease campaigning in Africa, for example, has utilized street theatre as a more effective means of communication with illiterate people than the more formal written door drop. Groups such as the homeless or those in prisons or other institutions should also be considered. Cultural issues should also be kept in mind so that specific messages can be communicated where these might apply – for example, in the disposal of bodies or the funeral process.

13.10   Internal Communications

During a crisis situation, it is very easy to forget about communicating internally within your own organization. This should be an integral part of a communications strategy ahead of a pandemic, to ensure that all the channels of communication are in place and those responsible know what to communicate to staff and when. Internal communications are a function that is sometimes the responsibility of the public relations or media team and sometimes a function of a human resources team. Whoever the responsibility sits with, it is crucial that staff are aware of how the organization will function during a pandemic and what arrangements there are for staff in terms of home working and carer's leave, etc. If the organization itself is heavily involved in working on an aspect of the pandemic, it is also useful for staff who are not working primarily in that area to be kept informed about what the organization itself is doing.

Staff can be updated by a variety of means including an intranet site, newsletters, e-mails and briefings. Messages to staff will differ through the various phases, the same as information for the public, for example, in the early phases issues like home working and what will be expected of staff can be communicated, whereas during the recovery phase there may be messages about how the organization may take some time to return to a normal level of output.

Internal staff communication is particularly important if the organization is key to the response to the pandemic. In such cases, it is essential to remember that staff will have the same worries and concerns as the rest of the public. They can act as ambassadors for your organization and are a good way to get information out to the community and quash rumours. However, communicating with staff can be difficult when simultaneously trying to get across the complexity of messages to the public – 'stay at home if ill with pandemic influenza' – versus messages to staff – 'it's really important to come to work to keep the organization running if you are well'.

13.11   Conclusion

Planning ahead and having a strategy in place for your communications is as important a part of pandemic preparedness as all other aspects discussed in earlier chapters, and can make or break the response to a pandemic. It is, however, something that is often omitted, left to the last minute or given only cursory thought. Communications activity is something that can work exceptionally well when it is thought through and well planned and not just a knee-jerk reaction to a crisis. Good, solid communications planning is therefore essential to support the breadth of pandemic preparedness undertaken by an organization; the best laid plans can easily come unstuck without the communications routes to tell people about them, or to ensure that the public knows what they should be doing to help themselves during the pandemic.

13.12   Summary Points

- It is crucial to have a communications strategy in place ahead of any crisis like a pandemic. This will help to determine the audiences with whom you need to communicate, the messages and timing of message delivery, your spokespeople and the other organizations you will be working with.
- To ensure the public receive your messages and act upon them you must take time to prepare them well by writing them in simple non-technical language and using good sentence structure and grammar; try to anticipate difficult questions now.
- Use a variety of channels for your messages to ensure they reach a wide audience and are absorbed and remembered.
- Be prepared for the onslaught of media interest once a pandemic starts and ensure you build relationships and agreements with journalists ahead of the pandemic beginning.
- Do not forget about communicating internally in your organization. Staff are a crucial asset in terms of both delivery and communications; it is important that they know what the organization expects of them during this time.

Further Reading

Centers for Disease Control and Prevention (2009) *Pandemic influenza risk communications guidance.* http://www.pandemicflu.gov/news/rcommunication.html (accessed May 2009).

European Centres for Disease Control (2009) *Pandemic Influenza – Innovations-Communication.* http://ecdc.europa.eu/en/healthtopics/Pages/Pandemic_Influenza_Innovations_ Communications.aspx (accessed September 2009).

Department of Health (2008) *Catch it, Bin it, Kill it – Respiratory and hand hygiene campaign.* http://www.dh.gov.uk/en/Publicationsandstatistics/Publications/PublicationsPolicy AndGuidance/DH_080839 (accessed May 2009).

Elledge, B.L., Brand, M., Regens, J.L. and Boatright, D.T. (2008) Implications of public understanding of avian influenza for fostering effective risk communication. *Health Promotion Practice* 9(4 Suppl.), 54S–59S.

Gupta, R.K., Toby, M., Bandopadhyay, G., Cooke, M., Gelb, D. and Nguyen-Van-Tam, J.S. (2006) Public understanding of pandemic influenza, United Kingdom. *Emerging Infectious Disease* 12, 1620–1621.

E. Collins

Pan American Health Organization (2009) Risk and Outbreak Communication homepage. http://www.paho.org/english/AD/SMC_HomePage_Eng.htm (accessed May 2009).

Plain English Campaign (2009) Homepage. http://www.plainenglish.co.uk (accessed May 2009).

World Health Organization (2005) *WHO outbreak communication guidelines*. http://www.who. int/infectious-disease-news/IDdocs/whocds200528/whocds200528en.pdf (accessed May 2009).

14 Case Study 1: Port Health and International Health Regulations

D. HAGEN

14.1 Introduction

A future pandemic will begin in one discrete location, from which it will spread nationally and internationally. Many experts predict that the pandemic epicentre will be in South-east Asia, based on the behaviour of previous pandemics in 1957 and 1968, and the opportunities in this region for interspecies transmission of influenza viruses; however, this is far from certain. Based on historical data, spread from the epicentre to neighbouring countries is expected to be swift, and data from the outbreak of severe acute respiratory syndrome (SARS) in 2003 and modelling studies both suggest that international travel (especially air travel) will facilitate rapid dissemination of the disease on a global scale. It is intuitive and instinctive to consider whether the spread of disease worldwide could be interrupted or delayed through travel-related countermeasures such as border controls, screening and forced reductions in international travel. While it is clear that these measures are highly unlikely to succeed, alone or in combination (see Chapter 10), even the idea of successful travel-related countermeasures inevitably draws attention to international ports and how port health functions should be handled during a pandemic. Although there is an inevitable focus on how port health issues will be used to handle the first few cases of pandemic influenza introduced into a country from outside its borders, the more relevant reality is that once pandemic influenza has established within a country's borders (i.e. is transmitting in the resident community) then control measures at ports will definitely have no further effect on the course of the pandemic within the country. For example, once pandemic influenza has entered a community, coming into contact with someone with symptoms on board an aircraft will have no greater relevance than coming into contact with someone with symptoms on a local bus.

Nevertheless, handling issues at ports will continue throughout the pandemic. Although international travel is expected to decline sharply during the pandemic period as people spontaneously change their behaviour and contact patterns, it will not cease completely; there is a natural instinct to 'return home' during a crisis and some international business travel will continue. Thus, passengers with influenza symptoms are still likely to present at ports (arriving and departing) and will need to be dealt with appropriately. It is also possible that 'health tourism' may encourage citizens from one country to attempt to cross into another because pandemic treatments (e.g. the availability of hospital care, antiviral drugs and vaccines) may be more readily available or cheaper.

©CAB International 2010. *Introduction to Pandemic Influenza*
(eds J.S. Nguyen-Van-Tam and C. Sellwood)

14.2   International Health Regulations (2005)

To understand the foundation upon which a response to a case of pandemic influenza at a port is to be planned, we must first examine the International Health Regulations (IHR). The World Health Organization (WHO) issued its first set of regulations intended to prevent the spread of diseases in 1951. They concentrated on only six 'quarantinable' diseases – cholera, plague, relapsing fever, smallpox, typhus and yellow fever – and were called the International Sanitary Regulations. These were renamed the International Health Regulations in 1969 and other public health issues have since appeared as international concerns. For example, three fundamental principles have been incorporated into the latest version of IHR:

1. Replacing the list of specific diseases with more generic illness.
2. Including chemical, biological and radiological agents as well as infectious agents.
3. Making some incidents notifiable within 24 h to the WHO if they fulfil the criteria to constitute a Public Health Emergency of International Concern (PHEIC – pronounced '*fake*'). PHEICs are reported through a National Focal Point for each of the 194 member countries.

In addition, the emphasis for member states has changed from control at borders to containment at source for international threats. This is consistent with the stated intention of the IHR:

> ...prevent, protect against, control and provide a public health response to the international spread of disease in ways that are commensurate with and restricted to public health risks, and which avoid unnecessary interference with international traffic and trade.

14.3   International Organizations

There are three primary organizations that advise the international air travel industry on public health and other issues, and hence response to an influenza pandemic:

1. The International Civil Aviation Association (ICAO), which represents its contracting countries and whose responsibilities are at country level.
2. The Airports Council International (ACI), which represents its individual airports.
3. The International Air Transport Association (IATA), which is a trade association representing the airline industry worldwide.

Each has developed contingency plans and guidelines for their respective areas of responsibility, most of which are available on the Internet and are well worth examining.

14.4   Misconceptions of Risk

There is a mistaken belief among the travelling public, often reinforced by public health officials, that if one person on board an aircraft has suffered from an infectious disease then all the remaining passengers are at high risk of acquiring that infection. There is little evidence to support this view, and in addition there are clear guidelines to follow in the event of incidents of infectious disease on aircraft among crew or passengers to mitigate any such incident. Although influenza transmission has been documented on board an airliner in Alaska (when the aircraft was grounded, the ventilation switched off and passengers were free to walk about), there are few other examples of transmission of confirmed influenza in such situations. Even this, often quoted example, may well have been due to transmission before or after the flight.

14.5   Lessons Provided by Severe Acute Respiratory Syndrome

Those planning for a public health response to an influenza pandemic often look at the international response to the SARS outbreak in 2003 for lessons.

SARS demonstrated just how rapidly the international spread of disease can occur in the modern age of air travel. From first appearing in Guangdong Province of southern China in November 2002, it only took 4 months to spread to 26 countries, causing nearly 800 deaths and over 8000 cases of infection. Transmission was facilitated by a Chinese doctor, who had treated patients with the 'unknown' respiratory illness, flying to Hong Kong and infecting others, as well as failures in isolation and infection control measures in healthcare facilities as far afield as Toronto in Canada.

SARS is a milestone with regard to air travel for several reasons:

- It was a newly emerging global threat first recognized only recently.
- It spread rapidly to more than two dozen countries in North America, South America, Europe and Asia before the outbreak was contained.
- It was spread readily by close contact.
- It was more amenable than influenza to proactive efforts due to the fact that peak infectivity occurred well after symptoms began and the incubation period was relatively long (3–10 days).
- General infection control precautions were the suggested actions (see Chapter 5 for more information).

Much publicity was given to exit screening in affected countries, both by medical questionnaire and thermal imaging, but these proved disruptive, ineffective and costly, requiring individual and public health action for febrile people.

According to flight schedule provider OAG, the number of scheduled flights worldwide fell by 3% – equivalent to 2.5 million seats – in mid-June 2003 compared with the same period in 2002. Flights to and from China showed a 45% drop in passenger numbers and the outbreak is estimated to have cost the world's airlines and travel-related industries approximately US$40 billion. Furthermore, the public's perception of risk of in-flight transmission of disease was influenced, despite the lack of evidence for this.

14.6   Travel Restrictions

Widely accepted modelling suggests that a 90% restriction on European air travel would delay the peak of a pandemic by only 1–2 weeks. Restrictions on travel from specific locations, for instance South-east Asia, would also be ineffective given the indirect flows of people from Asia to the rest of the world, as well as flows of people who would rapidly become infected in outbreaks in other countries (see Chapters 7

D. Hagen

and 10). Although there was a study in 2006 indicating that restricting air travel to the USA might have some domestic effect, most planners still accept the findings of a WHO technical consultation, which was held in Geneva in 2004 and attended by more than 100 experts from 33 countries, that stated:

> Providing information to domestic and international travelers (risks to avoid, symptoms to look for, when to seek care) is a better use of health resources than formal screening. Entry screening of travelers at international borders will incur considerable expense with a disproportionately small impact on international spread, although exit screening should be considered in some situations.

However, there will be intense political pressure to strengthen port health vigilance and implement restrictions in the early stages of the pandemic.

14.7   The Layered Approach

Both North America and the UK have adopted what is termed a 'layered approach' to port health, whereby several levels of response overlap and complement each other. This approach is necessary in an influenza pandemic as it is likely that: (i) the causes of influenza-like illness in passengers will be varied; (ii) asymptomatic infected individuals will not be detected by screening; and (iii) some travellers who are asymptomatically incubating the illness at the start of a long-haul flight may develop symptoms en route. The layered approach divides the actions into those at pre-embarkation, en route and upon arrival at the destination airport. Pre-embarkation measures may include:

- medical assessment of fitness to fly;
- screening by check-in or gate staff supported by airline-contracted, ground-based medical support (routine at present);
- self-administered medical questionnaire with assessment;
- questioning of passengers by trained staff; and
- thermal imaging.

Pre-embarkation measures would be applied throughout the pandemic but, as with most measures outlined here, the real value is in the early pandemic period before cases are found within a country. Early on, identification of cases will be a high priority given the enormous implications of a confirmed case and will be facilitated by rapid or near-patient tests when they become available. The real value in identifying cases before or once the virus is isolated in the country is to offer prophylaxis to those caring for the traveller and 'contacts' of the case, as well as for surveillance purposes. This would be of little value once outbreaks begin to occur within the country.

14.8   Generic Communicable Disease Control Applied to Pandemic Influenza

En route generic measures include enforcing existing IATA guidelines on dealing with suspected communicable diseases. These facilitate appropriate action in recognizing and dealing with any passenger fulfilling the criteria stated. Implementing these guidelines should give cabin crew the confidence to avoid over-reaction, such as the removal of a 16-year-old girl from a flight from Hawaii to New York due to an acute episode of coughing in March 2007.

IATA guidelines indicate that cabin crew obtain contact details from all travellers seated in the same row, two rows in front and two rows behind the sick traveller, utilizing Passenger Locator Cards. These cards were developed by the WHO to obtain public health contact tracing information and have been adapted for use by airlines and public health authorities internationally. Obtaining passenger data through airline manifest information continues to be problematic due to the nature of the details held by airlines, which are for financial purposes, and also because of confidentiality issues. In addition to the above measures, in July 2007 the ICAO introduced a system to provide earlier warning of public health events that would increase the window for mounting a public health response by reporting suspected cases of communicable disease via air traffic control services.

Despite evidence from the SARS response showing lack of effectiveness, arrival measures may include consideration of thermal imaging as a screening method, utilizing newer-generation equipment and/or having public health staff perform assessments on self-administered questionnaires completed upon landing or en route. Current generic arrival measures rely on isolation, which is the separation and restriction of movement of ill and potentially infectious individuals. Quarantine is the separation and restriction of movement of persons who, while not yet ill, have been potentially exposed to a communicable disease. It would require a large investment in resources to staff, accommodate and supply basic day-to-day needs in a secure area. This would require each country to pass legislation to ensure compliance and enforcement; and would also require a policy in place for removal of quarantine through near-patient or rapid testing or evidence-based clinical assessment. Neither isolation nor quarantine measures at ports would have any impact on population spread once cases of pandemic influenza had already been reported within a country.

14.9   Management of Pandemic Influenza at Ports

Management of pandemic influenza at ports of entry and exit to a country will require the cooperation of a myriad of organizations involved in the travel industry, as well as close liaison between public health and healthcare service providers. The greatest call on resources will occur early in the pandemic when there will be political pressure to be seen to be protecting the country from disease, despite the lack of evidence to support control measures.

Symptomatic individuals may need to be sent to hospitals or assessment centres for further investigation, and where possible these should be located near the airport. Early in the pandemic antivirals for cases and contacts may be available at ports but this facility would be quickly overwhelmed. Quarantine would require pre-arrangement of facilities which could provide all accommodation requirements as well as security to prevent escape and entry, as well as a predetermined endpoint to the application.

Any arrangements made at ports will require mechanisms to minimize direct contact with passengers and crew who may be subject to public health intervention, yet still satisfy security and immigration requirements. Table 14.1 summarizes the range of possible port health actions during a pandemic and the stages at which these might be most relevant to consider.

Table 14.1. Potential measures at ports at different stages of an influenza pandemic.

Measures	Pandemic declared	Virus isolated in country	Outbreaks within country	Widespread activity in country	Declining numbers	Comments
Information to travellers						
Details about the outbreaks	+	+	+	+	+	Full information on outbreaks must be shared
Advice, e.g. avoid non-essential travel	+	+	+	+	+	Country should issue advice early in pandemic
Repatriation (citizens and dead bodies)	–	?	?	–	–	Each country will have its own policy, but practicalities are immense
Border closures	–	–	–	–	–	No evidence to support
Port closures	–	–	–	–	–	Impractical
Pre-embarkation measures						
Medically fit to fly	+	+	+	+	+	Current practice
Screening at check-in	+	+	+	+	+	Current practice
Self-administered questionnaire	+	+	–	–	–	Early only
Questioning by trained staff	+	+	–	–	–	Supports above
Thermal imaging	?	?	–	–	–	No evidence to support
En route measures						
IATA guidelines – generic						
Identify sick passengers	+	+	+	+	+	Current practice
Infection control measures	+	+	+	+	+	Current practice
Consult ground-based support	+	+	+	+	+	Current practice
Advise port health	+	+	+	+	+	Current practice
Passenger locator cards	+	+	–	–	–	May be impractical later

continued

Table 14.1. Continued.

Measures	Pandemic stage					Comments
	Pandemic declared	Virus isolated in country	Outbreaks within country	Widespread activity in country	Declining numbers	
Arrival measures						
Thermal imaging	?	?	–	–	–	No evidence to support
Self-administered questionnaires	+	+	–	–	–	Useful early
Assessment by medical staff	+	+	–	–	–	Supports above
Isolation	+	+	+	+	+	Current practice, but unlikely to prevent population spread once cases are occurring within country
Quarantine	?	?	–	–	–	No evidence and impractical

IATA, International Air Transport Association.
Key: + = consider as potentially beneficial; – = not useful at this stage of the pandemic; ? = currently not supported.

D. Hagen

Further Reading

Airports Council International (2009) *Airport Preparedness Guidelines for Outbreaks of Communicable Disease.* http://www.airports.org/aci/aci/file/ACI_Priorities/Health/Airport%20 preparedness%20guidelines.pdf (accessed May 2009).

International Air Transport Association (2008) *Suspected communicable disease: general guidelines for cabin crew.* http://www.iata.org/NR/rdonlyres/DD29D97F-0E8C-4CBD-B575-1F5067174941/0/Guidelines_cabin_crew_May2009.pdf (accessed May 2009).

International Air Transport Association (2009) *Emergency Response Plan: A Template for Air Carriers, Public Health Emergency.* http://www.iata.org/NR/rdonlyres/1D412DF9-289B-4508-BE9D-A57C4A84F103/0/AirlinesERPChecklists_V1_Nov30.pdf (accessed May 2009).

International Civil Aviation Association (not dated) *Guidelines for States Concerning the Management of Communicable Disease Posing a Serious Public Health Risk.* http://www.icao.int/icao/en/med/AvInfluenza_guidelines.pdf (accessed May 2009).

Leder, K. and Newman, D. (2005) Review: Respiratory infections during air travel. *Internal Medicine Journal* 35, 50–55.

Moser, M.R., Bender, T.R., Margolis, H.S., Noble, G.R., Kendal, A.P. and Ritter, D.G. (1979) An outbreak of influenza aboard a commercial airliner. *American Journal of Epidemiology* 110, 1–6.

World Health Organization (2004) *WHO Consultation on priority public health interventions before and during an influenza pandemic, Geneva, 16–18 March 2004.* http://www.who.int/csr/disease/avian_influenza/pandemicconsultation/en/ (accessed May 2009).

World Health Organization (2005) *The International Health Regulations.* http://www.who.int/topics/international_health_regulations/en/ (accessed May 2009).

World Health Organization (2006) *Public health passenger locator card.* http://www.who.int/ihr/travel/locator_card/en/ (accessed May 2009).

15 Case Study 2: Issues Facing Pandemic Preparedness in Asia–Pacific Countries

L.C. Jennings

15.1   Introduction

The Asia–Pacific region plays a pivotal role in the epidemiology of both seasonal and pandemic influenza. The region is unique from the geographical perspective, as it encompasses countries from India to China, which contain approximately 52% of the global population of 6.5 billion people. The region also spans a full range of climates, from the northern temperate, through equatorial tropical, to southern temperate and includes both continental and island nations. These population and geographical characteristics support the continual circulation of seasonal influenza viruses and is believed facilitate the emergence of new human influenza variants. The region is also postulated to be the epicentre for the emergence of novel pandemic strains.

Although substantial progress has been made in pandemic preparedness planning in the region, with government commitment by most countries, the geographical immensity of the region, the size of the population and cultural and other issues, present challenges to ongoing planning.

15.2   Understanding the Burden of Influenza

The burden of influenza is poorly understood in countries in the tropical or subtropical zones where influenza activity is either poorly defined or is less pronounced than in temperate zones (see Chapter 1); this is due in part to continual virus circulation. The reasons for this often include the numerous competing infectious disease priorities, the lack of influenza surveillance, limitations of the public health infrastructure and the countries' socio-economic status.

Laboratory capacity building and influenza surveillance initiatives supported by the World Health Organization (WHO) and US Centers for Disease Control and Prevention (CDC) collaborative agreements since 2004, as well as burden of disease studies, are providing the necessary virological data and helping to reinforce the importance of influenza as a human disease in the region. However, in a number of countries in the region affected by A/H5N1, the focus has been largely on dealing with the ever-evolving A/H5N1 epizootic, particularly avian outbreak control and associated human infections, with pandemic preparedness planning somewhat further off and focused on strategic vision and the strengthening of future response capacity. This undoubtedly reflects the unique and difficult issues that these affected countries face, including limited financial and technical resources. In contrast, in countries where the seasonality of human influenza is well recognized (largely in the temperate zones), comprehensive

©CAB International 2010. *Introduction to Pandemic Influenza*
(eds J.S. Nguyen-Van-Tam and C. Sellwood)

pandemic plans are in place with detailed operational responsibilities clearly defined and implementation strategies utilizing the resources available described.

Clearly, an ongoing focus on surveillance and an increased understanding of the burden of disease associated with seasonal/human influenza are needed to ensure that pandemic preparedness planning is ongoing in the region. The WHO and non-government organizations such as the Asia–Pacific Advisory Committee on Influenza (www.apaci-flu.org), which has a focus on influenza awareness education, are key organizations in the region for ensuring this.

15.3 Pharmaceutical Measures (Availability of Antivirals and Vaccines)

The WHO has encouraged health authorities to consider stockpiling antiviral drugs; however, of the 40 countries globally with stockpiles of neuraminidase inhibitors, only seven of these are in the Asia–Pacific region. These stockpiles are all in middle-to high-income countries with dose numbers sufficient to treat between 5 and 43% of their populations. The existence of a WHO stockpile for a rapid containment response to an emerging influenza virus and increasing global availability of antivirals are unlikely to solve access issues for many countries in the region.

It is generally accepted that many countries, especially poor-resource/low-income countries, will need to confront the next pandemic with few or no vaccines. A number of countries are considering stockpiling human A/H5N1 vaccines. Of the eight countries with established stockpiles of human A/H5N1 vaccine, only two of these are in the Asia–Pacific region. Again, both are in middle- to high-income countries with vaccine doses sufficient to cover 2.4% and 16% of their populations, respectively. Even if pre-pandemic vaccines become more widely available, or alternatively vaccine manufacturing facilities are established in the region that are capable of producing pandemic vaccine, logistical issues of timely distribution and administration remain.

The countries with stockpiles of either neuraminidase inhibitors or human A/H5N1 vaccines all have pandemic plans and most have government recommendations in place for the use of seasonal influenza vaccines. Clearly, increasing government awareness of the importance of seasonal influenza, beyond the risk to travellers to the Hajj and the associated burden, is a key step towards integrated national influenza control strategies.

15.4 Non-pharmaceutical Measures (Use of Public Health Interventions)

Social distancing and personal hand and respiratory hygiene may be the only interventions available in many parts of the Asia–Pacific region. Although the evidence for the effectiveness of these measures is limited and is often based on mathematical modelling, they can be implemented at low cost. A number of countries have built on their experience during the outbreak of severe acute respiratory syndrome (SARS) in 2003 and have public personal hygiene education programmes in place. Some of these promote respiratory hygiene and hand washing among schoolchildren (e.g. the

SneezeSafe programme in New Zealand; www.sneezesafe.co.nz). Others have focused on healthcare providers rather than the general public for reasons such as fear of causing undue 'public concern', although public health web sites are widely available to all. Regardless, unless basic hygiene messages are publicized as a core management strategy for pandemic influenza, with preparations in advance to address the diverse cultural backgrounds and languages, they will be difficult to implement at the time of a pandemic alert (see Chapter 13).

The WHO places little emphasis on border management, except for island nations. However, many countries in the Asia–Pacific region are island nations, and their best protection from a novel influenza virus may be border management. The mortality during the 1918 pandemic was significantly higher in some of the poorly resourced countries in the region. It is not widely recognized that, following the entry of the 1918 virus into the Pacific island of Western Samoa in September 1918, 22% of the population died. In comparison, island countries where entry of the 1918 virus was delayed through the maintenance of strict border quarantine measures fared considerably better. The recognition of the importance of border management underpins both the Australian and New Zealand pandemic preparedness plans, where their phased response strategy is to delay the entry of any novel pandemic strains in the first instance.

15.5 Pandemic Exercises

The region has a track record for practising for the next pandemic. New Zealand was one of the first countries to test its pandemic plan by holding a national pandemic exercise (VIREX) in 2002, while Exercise Cumpston 06, held in Australia in 2006, was the largest ever government exercise in that country. Exercising is pivotal for the development of core pandemic preparedness infrastructure and expertise in countries because it allows government health authorities to work with the healthcare sector, border authorities and other agencies in a non-threatening environment (see Chapter 6). Even small desk-top exercises allow the dissemination of positive information to healthcare professionals and the public in a period of developing 'pandemic fatigue'.

15.6 Conclusions

Pandemic preparedness issues in the region are immense, however, with the ongoing commitment to pandemic planning by the WHO and financial support by donors, the commitment by individual governments is likely to be sustained. Influenza control strategies need to be developed or enhanced that involve surveillance and influenza awareness education. A focus on the development of surveillance capability is essential to ensure the early detection of both animal and human cases due to a novel influenza virus, allowing early containment, a critical step in most countries pandemic plan in the region. While general education on the seriousness of seasonal influenza will lead to the introduction and acceptance of prevention and treatment guidelines, the increased use of seasonal influenza vaccines will assist influenza vaccine availability during the next pandemic.

Further Reading: International Case Studies

Asia–Pacific Advisory Committee on Influenza (2007) National influenza pandemic plans. *Influenza – Asian Focus* (3), 4–5; available at http://www.apaci-flu.org/apaci/Activities-outputs/InfluenzaAsianFocus/tabid/59/Default.aspx (accessed January 2009).

Bell, D.M.; WHO Writing Group (2006) Non-pharmaceutical interventions for pandemic influenza, national and community measures. *Emerging Infectious Diseases* 12, 88–94.

Coker, R. and Mounier-Jack, S. (2006) Pandemic influenza preparedness in the Asia-Pacific region. *Lancet* 368, 886–889.

Jennings, L. (2005) New Zealand's preparedness for the next influenza pandemic. *New Zealand Medical Journal* 118, U1343.

Jennings, L.C., Monto, A.S., Chan, P.K.S., Szucs, T.D. and Nicholson, K.G. (2008) Stockpiling pre-pandemic influenza vaccines: a new cornerstone of pandemic preparedness plans. *Lancet Infectious Diseases* 8, 650–658.

Johnson, N.P. and Mueller, J. (2002) Updating the accounts: global mortality of the 1918–1920 'Spanish' influenza pandemic. *Bulletin of the History of Medicine* 76, 105–115.

McLeod, M.A., Baker, M., Wilson, N., Kelly, H., Kiedrzynski, T. and Kool, J.L. (2008) Protective effect of maritime quarantine in South Pacific jurisdictions, 1918–19 influenza pandemic. *Emerging Infectious Diseases* 14, 468–470.

Rambaut, A., Pybus, O.G., Nelson, M.I., Viboud, C., Taubenberger, J.K. and Holmes, E.C. (2008) The genomic and epidemiological dynamics of human influenza A virus. *Nature* 453, 615–622.

Russell, C.A., Jones, T.C., Barr, I.G., Cox, N.J., Garten, R.J., Gregory, V., Gust, I.D., Hampson, A.W., Hay, A.J., Hurt, A.C., de Jong, J.C., Kelso, A., Klimov, A.I., Kageyama, T., Komadina, N., Lapedes, A.S., Lin, Y.P., Mosterin, A., Obuchi, M., Odagiri, T., Osterhaus, A.D., Rimmelzwaan, G.F., Shaw, M.W., Skepner, E., Stohr, K., Tashiro, M., Fouchier, R.A. and Smith, D.J. (2008) The global circulation of seasonal influenza A (H3N2) viruses. *Science* 320, 340–346.

Oshitani, H., Kamigaki, T. and Suzuki, A. (2008) Major issues and challenges of influenza pandemic preparedness in developing countries. *Emerging Infectious Diseases* 14, 875–880.

World Health Organization (2005) *Avian influenza: assessing the pandemic threat*. http://www.who.int/csr/disease/influenza/H5N1-9reduit.pdf (accessed May 2009).

World Health Organization (2008) *Options for the use of human H5N1 influenza vaccines and the WHO H5N1 vaccine stockpile*. WHO Scientific Consultation, Geneva, Switzerland, 1–3 October 2007. http://www.who.int/csr/resources/publications/WHO_HSE_EPR_GIP_2008_1d.pdf (accessed May 2009).

World Health Organization Western Pacific Region (2008) *A Practical Guide for Designing and Conducting Influenza Disease Burden Studies*. http://www.wpro.who.int/NR/rdonlyres/68608B77-891B-4B36-B21D-F49E526E0B28/0/GuideforDesigningandConductingInfluenzaStudies.pdf (accessed May 2009).

World Health Organization (2009) *Epidemic and Pandemic Alert and Response (EPR)*. National Influenza Pandemic Plans. http://www.who.int/csr/disease/influenza/nationalpandemic/en/index.html (accessed May 2009).

World Health Organization (2009) *Epidemic and Pandemic Alert and Response (EPR)*. Pandemic Influenza Preparedness and Response. http://www.who.int/csr/disease/influenza/pipguidance2009/en/index.html (accessed June 2009).

16 Case Study 3: Issues Facing Pandemic Preparedness in Newly Independent States of the Former Soviet Union

SH. ARIPOV

16.1 Introduction

After the collapse of the Soviet Union in the last decades of the 20th century, all former Soviet Union (FSU) countries inherited a public health infrastructure based on the soviet sanitary-epidemiology model. Within this system considerable emphasis was placed on mandatory surveillance systems for infectious diseases, along with an emphasis on sanitary interventions (focused on disinfection and hygiene measures) coupled to strong vertical control from central government down towards regional and local levels. However, in the aftermath of the collapse of the soviet system this central coordination was lost, especially between countries, and resources were not always prioritized towards the development or maintenance of the existing public health infrastructure. Many FSU countries have relatively low socio-economic status and are undergoing a period of rapid economic reform and infrastructure rebuilding. Therefore there are numerous competing priorities for available development monies. In terms of pandemic preparedness activities, this lack of resources has delayed progress in many of the newly independent states compared with developed countries of the Western world. Nevertheless, it should be borne in mind that the remains of the former soviet system provide a strong framework and common configuration between the newly independent states, which can, in theory, produce many advantages in terms of coordinated action across more than one country in the region. There is a great need to coordinate activities and share pandemic preparedness information between countries in the region, however, independence has also created inter-country communication challenges that need to be resolved.

Several countries of the FSU, particularly the Central Asian republics, have already experienced outbreaks of highly pathogenic avian influenza (HPAI) A/H5N1 in poultry, which in some cases were associated with sporadic human cases, thus emphasizing the importance of avian influenza and its pandemic potential. Although not itself a part of the FSU, Turkey has also experienced HPAI A/H5N1 disease in birds and man and is an important trading partner and nearest neighbour in 'Europe' for many of the Central Asian countries; Istanbul also provides a major international air travel hub for most of Central Asia. The presence of HPAI A/H5N1 in Turkey has also driven considerable concern about its potential impact on poultry and man, and emphasized the importance of avian influenza control strategies (such as culling and disinfection). Paradoxically this has caused considerable misunderstanding about pandemic influenza, which is often misused as an alternative or interchangeable term for avian influenza. As a consequence, an all too commonly held view in the FSU is

©CAB International 2010. *Introduction to Pandemic Influenza*
(eds J.S. Nguyen-Van-Tam and C. Sellwood)

that pandemic influenza will definitely originate from an HPAI A/H5N1 virus and can be mitigated by control strategies associated with border controls, quarantine, disinfection, and controlling contact between wild and domestic birds. This view can be widely held among health professionals, public health workers and Ministry of Health officials, since the majority of personnel have not yet been trained on the differences between avian and pandemic influenza and the need for different preparedness strategies for each of these diseases.

Most FSU countries have now developed at least a first draft of a national pandemic plan; however, in many cases, the arrangements for implementation of strategic policies still require further development. This is also the case in many developed countries and represents a logical 'next step' in the evolution of pandemic preparedness after the preparation of national plans.

16.2   International Assistance

Significant levels of international assistance have been provided for avian influenza control and pandemic influenza preparedness within the region. Major donors such as the US Agency for International Development, the World Bank, the Asian Development Bank and the World Health Organization (WHO) support activities related to pandemic preparedness in FSU countries. However, even among these projects there is still confusion about the differences between avian influenza and pandemic influenza. For example, even though some projects are officially declared to be targeted at 'avian influenza control and pandemic influenza preparedness', they are nevertheless mainly focused on avian influenza control activities with far less attention to pandemic preparedness. This emphasizes the need to improve understanding and coordination of activities across the various donor agencies, and the need to make a clearer separation between avian influenza control and true pandemic preparedness.

16.3   Understanding the Burden of Influenza

The FSU countries have systems of communicable disease surveillance based on common soviet roots. Most systems are vertically controlled; clinical and laboratory data gathered at district level are delivered daily to regional centres where they are compiled and reported onwards to the Sanitary Epidemiological Surveillance Department (the precise name of this department varies between countries) within the Ministry of Health at national level.

Laboratory surveillance is performed on an ad hoc basis in some FSU countries and in selected areas in others. This activity is often limited by a lack of resources for purchasing modern equipment, consumables and reagents, and often depends on the resources provided by international donor agencies. In addition, laboratories in many parts of Central Asia do not have well-established practical mechanisms or the correct legislative framework for sending virus isolates to reference laboratories in other countries. Laboratory capacity building and influenza surveillance initiatives supported by the WHO, the World Bank and the US Centers for Disease Control and Prevention are helping to reinforce the importance of influenza as a human disease in the region. However, the importance of diagnosing human cases of A/H5N1 has again overemphasized the role of sophisticated diagnostic tests in pandemic preparedness, when in fact relatively few diagnostic tests will be performed or needed once a pandemic is established. The burden of influenza is still fairly poorly defined in countries and seasonal influenza vaccines are hardly used in some countries.

16.4 Pharmaceutical Measures (Availability of Antivirals and Vaccines)

The majority of FSU countries have very small quantities of neuraminidase inhibitors stockpiled for avian influenza and pandemic preparedness. This is partially due to the initial misunderstandings about the differences between avian influenza and pandemic; relatively small quantities of these drugs would be required to control an avian influenza incident, compared with the very large quantities needed for population treatment. However, the main driver is scarcity of financial resources and competing government priorities (e.g. modernization and infrastructure development, the need to address other vaccine-preventable infections). No FSU country has yet procured human HPAI A/H5N1 vaccines that could be used prior to a pandemic (see Chapter 9).

16.5 Non-pharmaceutical Measures (Use of Public Health Interventions)

Social distancing and personal hygiene may be the only interventions available in many parts of the FSU, although preparations to implement these are not yet well advanced in most countries. The WHO places little emphasis on border management, because in general such measures are not expected to be effective or delay the spread of pandemic influenza by more than a few weeks. However, there is a strong pre-existing culture of border controls in all FSU countries; while it is important that undue reliance is not placed on these measures, paradoxically they may be relatively easy to implement compared, for example, with Western Europe.

16.6 Pandemic Exercises

All FSU countries have written plans for the management of avian influenza and almost all have conducted simulation exercises, focused on an avian influenza incident and involving multiple ministries (e.g. Ministries of: Health; Agriculture and Water Resources; Emergencies). However, few countries have yet conducted pandemic preparedness exercises of any significant scale. It seems most likely that these will be scheduled after national pandemic preparedness plans are completed.

16.7 International Health Regulations

All FSU republics are signatories to the International Health Regulations (IHR) (Chapter 14). Some countries (e.g. the Russian Federation) have internal State regulations (signed by the State Chief Sanitarian Physician in Russia) obliging all interested

S. Aripov

parties to participate in planning and implementation of the IHR in their countries. Capacity assessment and planning for the implementation of IHR in FSU countries is currently being undertaken and should be well underway by 2009. The majority of FSU republics participate in annual coordination meetings related to the IHR, information sharing and emergency preparedness, also organized by the WHO.

16.8 Conclusions

Pandemic preparedness is well underway in the newly independent states of the former Soviet Union. Most countries focused initially on the control of avian rather than pandemic influenza, because of the close geographical proximity of the HPAI A/H5N1 epizootic. However, this has created considerable misunderstanding, which has hampered the process of pandemic preparedness. This has now been resolved in many countries through the efforts of the WHO. Although many countries now have a national pandemic plan, there are many issues of considerable significance that remain. However, a strong framework and common configuration from the former soviet system remains across the newly independent states, which can, in theory, produce many advantages in terms of coordinated action as pandemic preparedness continues to evolve in the region.

Conclusion

A future influenza pandemic is inevitable, but its timing and intensity cannot be predicted. Three such events occurred in the last century, of which two were mild and one was extremely severe. Regardless of its severity, the next influenza pandemic is likely to produce a global public health emergency for which preparation in advance is a necessity. For the first time in human history specific influenza treatments will be available alongside traditional public health countermeasures. In addition, advances in vaccine technology have improved the chances of early access to vaccines and offered the possibility of pre-pandemic deployment strategies. Against these new advantages are set the additional problems of a world in which country interdependencies are greater than ever before, and international travel is so commonplace that very rapid spread is inevitable.

Previous human pandemics have been caused by A/H1, A/H2 and A/H3 subtypes. Credible pandemic threats currently exist from a range of avian influenza viruses, most notably A/H5N1, and A/H7 subtypes. It is totally impossible to predict the identity (subtype) of the next human pandemic virus or to attach meaningful numerical probability to the likelihood of a given subtype producing the next pandemic. Nevertheless, the current A/H5N1 epizootic and its worrying incursion into man has raised awareness and created a window of opportunity for advance preparation, which we must exploit to our advantage. Swine influenza A/H1N1 has also recently presented a second pandemic threat from a most unexpected direction, reinforcing our uncertainty about the origins of the next pandemic and the need to maintain worldwide vigilance.

All countries need to be as well prepared as possible, ensuring plans encompass not just health aspects but also wider business and community implications. This will help to ensure that the response to any future pandemic is as good as it possibly can be and takes advantage of the many technological, societal and medical developments of the last few years.

Index

infection: control *see under* control: of
 infection
information and communication 168
 challenges 190(box)
 communications team 182–183
 during recovery phase 188, 190
 importance 153, 183
 internal communications 191
 issues of public concern 183(box)
 local communications 190–191
 media 185–186
 spokespeople and trust 186–187
 timing and intensity 188
 varied strategy 187–188
 WHO principles for outbreak
  communication 184–185
institutions, closed and semi-closed
 8–9, 166
interdependencies 77
International Air Transport Association
 (IATA) 195
International Civil Aviation Association
 (ICAO) 195
International Health Regulations (WHO,
 2005) 195, 208–209
Internet 186
interoperability 77, 154–155

jargon 185

language: importance 184–185
leopards 32–33
litigation 161, 165
Lysovir® *see* amantadine

M2 inhibitors 20, 36, 98
 adverse events 100–101
 development and trials 99–100
 efficacy in treatment and prophylaxis
  100
 resistance 101
 site of action 99(fig)
M2 protein 20
marketing authorizations 125
masks, surgical 65–66, 67, 140–141(tab)
mass media 185–186
media (communication) 185–186
mice: as animal transmission model 64
migration, bird 30–31

mitigation 93–94(box), 151–152
'mock-up' vaccines 125
models and modelling
 animal models 64, 124
 biomathematical modelling
  of antiviral drug usage 109(box)
  assessment of pandemic severity
   88–89
  definition 87–88
  distancing and school closures
   150–151(box)
  economic models 92
  of interventions and
   countermeasures 89–90
  key papers 93–94(box)
  real-time 92, 94–95
  SIA and SIR models 90–92
  travel restrictions 149(box)
  UK Scientific Pandemic Influenza
   Committee Modelling
   Sub-Group 94(box)
  and vaccination strategies 131(box)
  value 96
morbidity 158–159
 and age 5, 51(box)
 psychiatric 159
 seasonal influenza 3
mortality 158
 A/H5N1 36
 and age 5
 age-specific 46(fig)
 excess deaths 6–7, 46–47
 seasonal influenza 3

neuraminidase inhibitors 21, 36, 98
 adverse events 104
 comparison 107(tab)
 development 101–102
 ease of use and stockpiling 105–107
 efficacy in treatment and prophylaxis
  102–103
 pharmacokinetics 102
 site of action 99(fig)
 viral resistance 104–105
nomenclature: influenza viruses 17–18
nosocomial infection 8–9

oseltamivir 36, 99(tab)
 active pharmaceutical ingredient (API)
  105–106